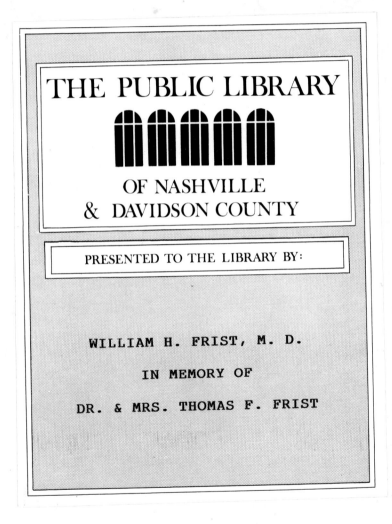

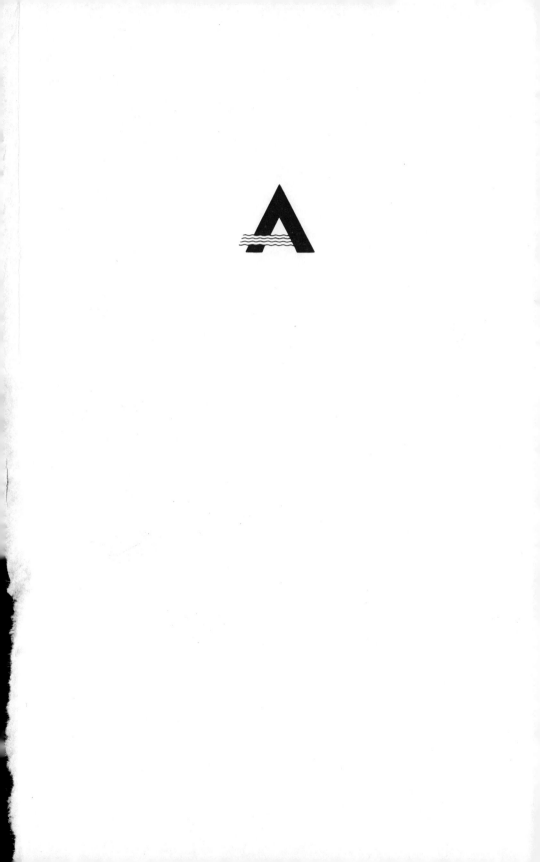

TRANSPLANT

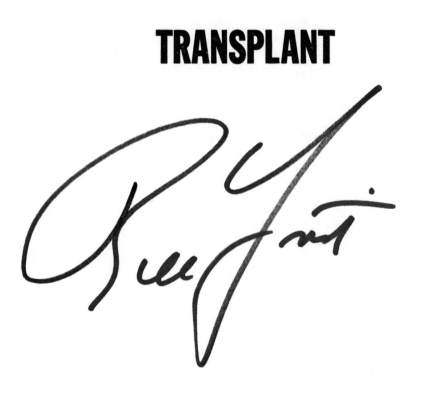

TRANSPLANT

*A Heart Surgeon's Account
of the Life-and-Death Dramas
of the New Medicine*

William H. Frist, M.D.

A MORGAN ENTREKIN BOOK
THE ATLANTIC MONTHLY PRESS
NEW YORK
·

Published simultaneously in Canada
Printed in the United States of America

Library of Congress Cataloging-in-Publication Data

Frist, William H.
    Transplant: a heart surgeon's account of the life-and-death
    dramas of the new medicine / William H. Frist.

    "A Morgan Entrekin book."
    ISBN 0-87113-322-9
    1. Heart—Transplantation—Popular works.   I. Title.
    RD598.F75 1989   89-30287   617'.4120592—dc19

Design by Laura Hough

The Atlantic Monthly Press
19 Union Square West
New York, NY 10003

FIRST PRINTING

For Karyn, Harrison,
Jonathan, and Bryan

Contents

Preface

This book covers a year in the heart-transplant program at Vanderbilt University Medical Center in Nashville, Tennessee. It is the story of one transplant surgeon's attempt to come to terms with his life—with the complex issues and vexing problems that abound in transplantation; with the heartrending and joyous adventures of the explorers known as transplant recipients; and with the needs and pleasures of a private life centered around a loving and supportive family.

This is not a journal, not a diary, not a true confession. It's a nonfiction narrative, with the emphasis on narrative. The form requires certain liberties. Wherever possible, I have used the actual names of those involved; occasionally, the delicate nature of a topic or my own sense of fairness has led me to omit a name entirely or disguise it in some fashion. There are, however, no invented characters. The conversations and dialogue are as I remember them or as they were reported to me, sometimes edited or "improved" in the interest of greater clarity and a larger truth. Similar considerations sometimes led me to telescope events, as historical dramatists often do. Nevertheless, what I portray did in fact happen, by and large as I report it. I think that's all that can be claimed for any work of nonfiction.

Hardly a day goes by without a newspaper or television report about a life saved by an organ transplant. That's what transplantation, one of the most remarkable success stories in the history of medicine, is all about: saving lives. And this book would not have been possible without the surgeons, physicians, nurses, transplant coordinators, immunologists, and pharmacologists, the medical pioneers who joined forces to make that success story possible and to bring new life—full and productive life—to the thousands and thousands of transplant recipients.

This book, however, is not for them. It is for those of all ages, all races, and all walks of life who wait anxiously for a new heart or heart and lungs. There is no need for a single one of those men and women and children to die. Yet as many as one in five will, simply because we do not have enough organs to go around. Today, heart transplantation is in the mainstream of American medicine. The number of heart transplants has risen tenfold in the past five years, and with this explosive growth come difficult questions: ethical issues of who should receive a new heart; religious and social issues about brain death; financial issues concerning equal access to the new medicine; political issues of allocation of scarce resources.

If a reader gets nothing else out of this book but the knowledge that there is a critical organ shortage in America and that he or she should at least think about becoming a donor, then my purpose will be served. My hope is, of course, that *all* those who read this book will decide to become organ donors and will make that decision clear to their loved ones.

To that end, let me tell you a few things you should know about organ donation:

- Organ donation does not affect or delay customary funeral arrangements.
- There is no cost to the family, nor is there any payment for donation; hospital expenses incurred prior to the donation of organs and funeral expenses remain the responsibility of the donor's family.
- Organ donation is consistent with the beliefs of all major religions.
- Individuals under the age of eighteen may sign a donor card with the consent of their parent or legal guardian.
- It is not necessary to mention organ donation in your will.

- If you wish to donate your body for anatomical study, you should contact a medical school in your community.
- Donor cards provided by various national and local organizations have the same validity as the one on your driver's license. You will be recognized as a donor anywhere in the United States as long as you sign and carry a donor card.
- All patients awaiting a transplant are registered on a national computer system, and when organs are donated, this system helps distribute them where they are most needed.
- One donor can help many recipients through the gift of different organs and tissues.
- Most organs and tissues can be stored for a limited time and can be transported to any location where they are needed; most likely, there is a hospital in your community doing transplants.
- Most importantly, the future of transplantation depends upon the support of people like you.

I did not make the journey described in the following pages alone, and I would like to thank those who traveled with me. Charles Phillips, a professional writer, collaborated with me in the telling of my story, guiding me through the intricacies of narrative even as I walked him through the world of a surgeon and introduced him to the complexities of transplantation. We not only survived, we both enjoyed the trip. I would also like to thank Kyle Young for providing the spark that brought Charlie and me together and Patricia Hogan for her careful reading of our various drafts.

My wife, Karyn, accompanied me not only through the telling of the story, but—what was infinitely more impressive— through the occasional pain of living it as well. Without Drs. Norman Shumway, Ed Stinson, Phil Oyer, and Vaughn Starnes, I could not even have begun the journey. Harvey Bender and especially Walter Merrill, my close friend whose approach to medicine should serve as a model for all future physicians, made my dreams reality. The dedication of transplant nurse Jan Muirhead, the institutional support of Vanderbilt and Vice-Chancellor Ike Robinson, and the inspiration of patients like Jim Hayes all contributed in their own powerful way to this story.

The journey simply could not have been made without the help of those I've mentioned. Writing a book, even when you are telling your own story, is very much like heart-transplant surgery in at least one important way: it's a team effort.

TRANSPLANT

Part One

MIDNIGHT RUN

1

Harrison, my four-year-old son, wanted a story.

He sat beside me, small and delicate, dressed in his blue-striped pajamas, ferociously turning the pages of his book, hoping we would forget that it was his bedtime.

He understood the signs: the ten o'clock news, the indulgent smiles on our faces, the subtle changes in our tones of voice. He seemed to think that somewhere, somehow he could find in his book precisely the magic formula that would hold off forever the voice of doom, the voice that now announced in no uncertain terms, "Harrison, it's time."

When he heard the words, he looked at his mother and knew he was a goner. Against hope, he pleaded, "But Daddy's going to read me a story."

As I lifted him up to climb the stairs and deliver on my earlier promise, I was struck by how much more he weighed than I remembered. I wondered if Bryan, the baby, had grown heavier, too, and Jonathan, our two-year-old. Bryan was already asleep when I got home from the hospital—when? An hour ago. And though my wife, Karyn, had tried to keep Jonathan awake so I could spend some time with him, he had collapsed on the floor of the den. I found him curled up under the glass coffee table. Only Harrison, who at four years old had joined the Frist family's hereditary war on sleep, showed the stamina needed to greet the shadowy figure he vaguely knew was his father.

I had missed their first steps, missed their discovery of the spoken word, missed most of their young lives. During my tenure as chief resident in cardiothoracic surgery at Stanford, I was often gone for two, sometimes three days, napping (if I slept at all) in the hospital, before I made it home to Karyn, the newborn

3

Jonathan, and the toddler Harrison. I was aware that other residents and interns had watched their marriages crack, their homes vanish, and their work suffer under the miserable assaults of guilt and resentment. I counted myself lucky. Karyn approached the situation as a challenge, managed the house and children alone, encouraged me in my work, and never made me feel guilty.

I swore I would not become like the others. I took refuge in the great respect I had for my wife and the sacrifices she made. I told myself that even occasional days with the children could make a difference if I took pains to ensure the time I spent with them was special. I remembered my father, also a physician, talking like that, and it had surely worked for him when I was young. But even now, years later, on those rare evenings when I was home long enough to see the boys, some little thing—the way one of my children treated a book, a new turn of phrase, a few extra pounds—would bring back the doubt. It seemed to me that my presence often disrupted their lives rather than enriched them, and I felt almost like an intruder.

The telephone rang. I had been reading to Harrison for only a few minutes, and I looked up with what I suspect was the same indignant expression he had flashed at Karyn when she told him to go to bed.

Karyn stood in the hallway, holding the phone.

"It's Rusty," she said.

"Rusty, what's up?" I looked at Karyn, and she turned away. Rusty was a coordinator for the organ-procurement agency in Nashville that served middle Tennessee. His call meant, she knew, that someone had died—suddenly, violently.

"I think we've got a heart," Rusty said. "Down in Florida. Just got off the phone with the coordinator there. Donor is blood type A, thirty-two-year-old male, 175 pounds, 5'10". You got someone?"

Jim Hayes, I thought. Jim was a very special patient. He'd had his first heart transplant years ago at Stanford, when heart-transplant surgery was still experimental and half of the patients died soon after the operation. (Over the years, heart-transplant care has improved dramatically. With the discovery of new techniques and drugs, ninety percent of all patients now survive.) Jim had beaten the odds in 1976. He had celebrated the fifth anniversary of his new life by bicycling from his home in Knoxville, Tennessee, to California for his annual checkup, in an effort to call attention to the miracle of transplantation. He had remarried, sired a son who became the center of his new life, and written a sensitive, insightful book about his experience.

Then, two years ago, his new heart began to develop atherosclerosis, the hardening of the arteries that causes most heart attacks. The disease ran rampant and destroyed his heart's underlying pumping function. At his last annual evaluation at Stanford, the transplant team told Jim that his only hope was to undergo a second transplant. Without it, he'd be dead in six months.

"The EEG's been flat since this morning," Rusty said. "They're about ready to declare the guy brain dead. Thought you'd like to know now, start going over your list."

"Cause of death?"

"Car accident. Two days ago. Wasn't wearing a seat belt, his head went through the windshield. They say he was unresponsive from the moment they brought him to the emergency room. He hasn't improved—no spontaneous activity off the ventilator. Wasn't carrying a donor card. The coordinator there just talked to the wife and brother, and they're willing to donate all the organs."

"They know how we want the body managed?"

"Yeah, I told them how we want the fluids handled and which antibiotics to give. There's a kidney team coming up from Miami. Bones and eyes are going locally. Apparently they couldn't find a match for the liver."

"Sounds good, Rusty. Let me look over my list. Give me a call as soon as the lab work is ready. Find out what his urine output and central pressures are. Say, fifteen minutes?"

"You got it."

When I hung up the phone, Karyn was watching me, her big, expressive eyes holding a sadness I could never afford to feel. These calls always upset her. I knew she was thinking about the

5

dead man I called a donor, wondering whether he had a wife and children, worrying about how they felt. I had learned early that if I wanted to be a transplant surgeon, I could not dwell on the futility and tragedy almost always associated with a donor's death. Brain death seemed to be death at its most unfair because it resulted so often from sudden, unexpected accidents or violence. Its victims were usually young, healthy people in their prime. Placed on ventilators, their bodies kept active courtesy of science and its machines, they even looked alive, appeared to breathe, seemed to be in a deep, peaceful sleep.

In fact, I thought grimly, that's just what made them good donors. I knew the way Rusty and I talked might seem ghoulish to some, but the truth was that my professional existence rested on the terrible paradox that someone had to die before my patients could be given the chance to live. My job was to save sick people, not worry about those who were already lost.

Still, there were Karyn's eyes.

"How did he die?" she asked, always her first question.

"Automobile accident," I said, hoping she'd stop there.

"Did he have a family?"

"I think so," I said, reaching quickly into my pocket for the three-by-five-inch card listing my patients waiting for hearts. I carried the card night and day. Every time I looked at it, I again became aware that at least two or three people listed there would die before I could find them new hearts. Not a month went by that I didn't lose a patient needlessly. It was unquestionably the most painful, most trying, and most disappointing part of my work.

It seemed truly unfair. Thousands of suitable organs were wasted every year because families simply did not know, had never been told that they had the chance to save lives, to pull hope from the wreckage, to find some consolation amidst their anguish. The deaths of their loved ones did not have to be totally in vain. I knew from my own experience, and the careful documentation of others, that donating the organs of a deceased loved one helped families through their grief.

Of the eight patients on my list, five needed hearts and three needed hearts and lungs. Only two—Jim Hayes and a man from

Madison, Tennessee—matched the body size and blood type of our donor. It was an agonizing decision, the kind I hate to make because I shouldn't have to. No one should, given the number of potential donors. The odds were that the man I chose would be alive ten years from now; the other would very possibly be dead in a month, his futile wait for a heart at an end. Jim Hayes had already had one donor heart; shouldn't we give this one to the Madison man? Finally, it was Jim Hayes's rapidly weakening condition that made up my mind.

"This may be Jim Hayes's lucky day," I said to Karyn.

I resisted the urge to call Jim immediately. There was still too much that could go wrong. Instead, I dialed Walter Merrill, my surgical associate, at home, woke him up, told him we might be doing a transplant later.

"Great!" he said, his voice thick with sleep yet edged with excitement. By the time we finished working out the preliminary logistics, Rusty was on the line again.

"The neurologist declared our boy brain dead minutes ago, and the liver and kidney functions are all normal. We're still waiting for the serologies for hepatitis and AIDS, but my guess is he's a low risk for either one. His urine output and blood pressure are okay, and he's on a very small dose of dopamine."

"Good. How's his fluid status?"

"The coordinator swears to me he's being rehydrated and weaned off the dopamine."

As Rusty talked, I worked over the problem in my mind. Our donor had smashed his head; the soft, almost mushy brain usually swells inside the rigid skull after it suffers severe trauma. Hoping to save the patient's life, the Florida trauma doctors had probably tried to reduce the swelling by dehydrating their patient and putting him on dopamine, which would make the heart pump harder, raise the patient's blood pressure, and keep blood flowing to the brain. But medicines like dopamine, known as inotropes or pressors, could damage the heart muscle if used to excess. Now that the doctors had declared the patient brain dead,

7

the coordinator would enter the picture and immediately attempt to rehydrate the donor by pumping fluid into his veins, raising his blood pressure naturally while weaning him off the dopamine. Dopamine could make even a bad heart pump deceptively well. The heart could be sluggish, even permanently damaged, and none of us would know it until they reduced the dosage.

"So far, it sounds ideal," I said. "I'd like to leave the hospital here by midnight. Can we do that?"

"Sure, I'll get right on it."

By the time I left for Vanderbilt Hospital, I had made a dozen other calls. I phoned Walter back to tell him we had a go, and I called to schedule an operating room.

"If we're on the way down there by twelve, I think we can count on cutting skin here about five in the morning. What do you think?"

"Sounds right," he said. "Would you rather me go to Florida?"

"No, that's OK. I'm already up and running."

We synchronized our watches, knowing that I would be in touch at least every thirty minutes during the next six hours. We had to time everything as precisely as possible, from my first look at the donor heart in Florida to the moment we stitched Jim Hayes together again back in Nashville.

I reached Jan Muirhead just as she was going to bed. Jan is a rail-thin clinical nurse specialist in heart transplantation and my right arm in dealing with transplant patients and their families. I called the hospital admitting officer to make sure we would have no paperwork delays in getting Jim onto the operating table. I called the operating room to confirm the surgery, to ask the nurses to have the cardioplegic solutions ready, and to prepare the necessary equipment for me to take to Florida. I called the cardiac recovery room to set up the isolation room where transplant patients are placed right after surgery. I paged Dr. Tom Wareing, the chief resident in Vanderbilt's cardiac surgery service, to tell him when Jim would arrive so he could meet him at the door and examine him as soon as possible. I rang the blood bank to request six units of packed red blood cells for the operation. I dialed Dr. Jim Atkinson, the transplant pathologist who would scoop up Jim's old heart as soon as we cut it out and examine it in the laboratory. I paged Dr. Ben Byrd, the Vanderbilt transplant team's cardiologist, our nonsurgical heart specialist.

And I called Jim Hayes to tell him we had found his new heart.

Sometime during all of this Karyn had gone to bed, and I had moved back down to the den to avoid disturbing her with the seemingly endless list of calls I had to make. Before I left for the hospital, I trooped back upstairs to say good-bye.

"Who's going to Florida?" She asked. "You or Walter?"

"I am," I said. "Maybe I can catch some sleep on the plane."

"Do you want me to cancel the babysitter for tomorrow night?"

"I guess you'd better. I don't think I'll be back from the hospital in time. I'm sorry."

"No. No, that's all right."

On the way out, I sneaked a last look at the boys. Harrison hadn't moved at all, it seemed, since I had left him lying there earlier, hugging my old teddy bear. I wondered how many times my own father had looked down at me, clinging to the same stuffed toy, before he took off in the middle of the night and drove to someone's home to sit, perhaps, by a bed and hold a dying patient's hand. Had he, too, tried to tell himself that his work justified being an absentee father and husband? Had he, too, occasionally heard the disappointment in Mother's voice, the way I had heard it in Karyn's just now? Did he, too, realize what an impossible life we asked them to live? Did he, too, wonder if the thrill of losing himself so totally in his profession grew from a burning desire to help others or from an overpowering need to keep a part of himself aloof, even from those he loved the most?

A doctor is a man whose job justifies everything. I had a Lear jet to catch and a heart to retrieve.

2

There's something about a hospital at night.

I find that there's a kind of solitude, a peacefulness, that's missing during the day, especially in an operating room. By their very nature, hospitals are intense places, where life and death battle constantly and the intensity feeds on the emotions of those thrown together in the struggle. In the daytime, the emotional intensity grates on the nerves. Patients have one set of problems, families another, nurses and doctors yet another. They—and social workers and administrators and the army of others—bump into one another, say hello, seek reassurance, ask a question, bark an order, and get on with their jobs. When you meet someone during the day, they're almost always on the way to somewhere else. The strain is in the air.

At night the intensity is still there, but it's shared by fewer people: it's focused. The struggle is quieter, calmer, almost solemn. I'm sure that part of the reason is that without the high-strung, stressful hustle, people are more relaxed, more themselves. I know I am. Maybe part of it is the bittersweet, secret pleasure of martyrdom, working late when the rest of the world is asleep or playing; it may even be a certain nostalgia for my days as a surgical resident in Boston, when the hospital was literally home for thirty-six of every forty-eight hours, year round. But I think it's more than all that; it's a mystical aura, something serene and magical.

I love a hospital late at night.

There was only one car in the parking garage; it had been sitting there for days. As I locked my door and made my way toward the office, the night watchman looked up from his station and nodded. He was a bizarre sight, dressed in a blue uniform and cap, his nostrils hooked to an oxygen tank behind his desk by two long green tubes. As a guard, he didn't exactly inspire confidence.

A former two-pack-a-day smoker with end-stage bronchitis, he had approached me shortly after I arrived from Stanford and asked about his chances for getting a lung transplant. He was too old, and he had the wrong kind of lung disease to qualify, but we all need hope. So I told him "maybe," "someday," "if our research pans out," and now he always wanted to talk. I stopped, chatted with him briefly, then darted off to my office to retrieve Jim Hayes's file.

Rusty caught up with me in the third-floor surgical wing.

"Ambulance is standing by downstairs, next to the emergency ward," he said. He tossed his thick donor-protocol journal on the bench in the men's dressing room as we put on our surgical scrubs. He pushed his sandy brown hair back out of his eyes, ran his fingers over his neatly clipped moustache, and flashed his friendly, upbeat smile.

"The Lear's ready," he said, "and I've arranged for a helicopter to meet us in Tampa. It'll be fifteen, twenty minutes by chopper to the hospital. Would've taken an hour, maybe, by ambulance." He paused. "Worries me that they've never handled a heart before. Small hospital. In the middle of nowhere."

"I know. Me too. Any more on the donor?"

"I've been in constant touch. They *say* everything is okay."

My beeper went off. There was a phone in the dressing room. Jim Hayes came on the line.

"Hi, Doc," he said. "How's it going? You said to call you when we got halfway there." I had not wanted him to drive all the way to Nashville if everything wasn't falling into place.

"That's good, Jim. That's good. Now you come on in and don't worry about a thing."

"I'm not worried, Dr. Frist, as long as you're not."

I didn't tell him that I was. There were so many details, so many things to go wrong with the donor heart, the transporta-

11

tion, the crossmatch. I had told him earlier, as I told all my patients, that unless absolutely everything fell into place, we'd call off the transplant. I might do it at any stage. There could be no shortcuts, no compromises. He could even be put to sleep, prepped, his body shaved, and we would wake him up, say we were sorry, send him home again for another long, terrible wait. That had happened to others. Now, I just tried to reassure him. And myself.

"Dr. Frist," Rusty said when I hung up. "This place is going to be pretty small. They probably won't have a chest retractor."

I stifled the urge to make him call the donor hospital one more time. Instead, I said, "Right. Why don't you go on downstairs and grab one while I look over the stuff up here."

On our way out, we ran into Nancy Davis. She was an organ-procurement coordinator who also worked for Rusty's outfit. Like a physician, she was on call twenty-four hours a day. Her hair was still wet, an inky outline to her features.

"I'm coming, I'm coming," she said and disappeared into the women's dressing room.

By the time Rusty got back upstairs and Nancy reappeared in her scrubs, I had looked over the supplies: two pairs of scissors; tubing and a pressure bag for the cardioplegic solutions that stop the heart just before we take it out; two big, clear plastic bags to put the heart in; a plastic container for the bags; six bags of saltwater solution to cool the heart down; and, of course, the red and white Igloo picnic cooler, the standard high-tech container for transporting a donor organ. I didn't know what the hospital near Tampa would have on hand—every hospital was different—but the idea was to keep things simple and use as many of their surgical instruments as possible. That way we didn't waste a lot of time trying to sort out our equipment from theirs at the end while the heart sat around dying in an ice chest.

"Let me call Walter," I said. "I'll tell him we're on our way."

At the elevators, a couple of nurses noticed the Igloo cooler. The petite blonde said, "Where you headed?"

"Florida," I said.

"Need another nurse?" the tall brunette said. "Promise I won't get in the way."

The elevator door closed on their "Good luck."

The midnight ambulance ride to the airport was quiet. We were doing well on time, and there was no need for sirens and breakneck speed—yet. Sometimes there was, and I often thought those rides were the most dangerous part of the whole procedure. "Transplant Team Dies in Ambulance Crash," the headline would read. Then there would be five hearts for someone else to harvest. Provided, of course, we had each signed donor cards, talked it over with our next of kin, and wound up in a hospital where the doctors routinely asked about donation, as federal law required.

Chances were that not all of those things would happen, even given who we were and what we were doing.

I sat in the back of the ambulance, looking at the empty stretcher opposite my seat and thinking about sleep. There were no windows, and in the lull and sway of the ride my mind grew fuzzy. I was up at five o'clock this morning, I thought. Home at midnight the night before. Five hours sleep in thirty-six. Weren't you the one waxing eloquent about the good old days as a resident? I glanced at Rusty and Nancy, both absorbed in their own thoughts, and drifted off.

Suddenly, automatically, I was alert again, reviewing our progress with the obsessiveness as essential to a transplant surgeon as manual dexterity. I forced myself to think through each step of the routine once we got to Florida, worried that I was taking something for granted, forgetting a detail, leaving something to chance. I couldn't do that. The smallest slip could be disastrous. Cost me a heart. A patient.

Our ambulance was cleared onto the airport runway, and I saw the sleek lines of the elegant flying machine poised and waiting for us, its pilot and copilot standing around in their conservative business suits.

"I feel like I'm wearing pajamas," Nancy said.

13

"I doubt they see many passengers as underdressed as we are," I said. We climbed aboard. The copilot helped us to get comfortable, pointed out the emergency exit and the place they stored the refreshments, and took his place in the cockpit. The pilot was already talking to the tower. Cleared for takeoff, within minutes we were taxiing down the runway lined with flashing strobes.

Small and swift, Lear jets spoil you for other travel. As we shot up to our cruising altitude of 31,000 feet and leveled off for the forty-minute flight, I settled back into the comfort of the sofa-sized seat and inhaled the rich perfume of fine leather. When the pilot turned off the cabin lights, I caught the pale fire of the full moon hung against a midnight-blue sky, Venus shining bravely by its side and the moonlight reflecting off the thick layer of clouds that stretched toward the horizon.

Mesmerized by the aching beauty of the night, I suddenly missed flying like a lost love. I longed for the sense of freedom it gave me, for the exhilaration of height and speed, for the blank and silent solitude of a vast sky. I had had my pilot's license since I was little more than a boy, logging hundreds of hours of flight time, taking to the air during college, medical school, and surgical residency whenever I felt a dreary November in my soul or the suffocating weight of routine. When I flew my little Apache and looked down at civilization, I felt powerful and insignificant at the same time; most importantly, I felt in control of my destiny. Flying was my big fix, the only way I knew to relax completely. It had been months since I had taken a plane up. The new transplant program at Vanderbilt had left little time for it. Since beginning the program a year before, I had flown perhaps three times.

"That's pretty good," Karyn would say. "More times than you made it home to dinner."

The clouds had prevented me from getting my bearings on the lights of Nashville as we headed south, prevented me from fixing the exact point where I lived, the house where Karyn and the boys were now fast asleep. But I searched below anyway, knowing that even if there had been no clouds, I couldn't have seen it; when I left, the house had been dark, a shadowy thing sitting up on the hill behind me as I had pulled out of the driveway. I hadn't picked out the house; I hadn't even seen it before I moved in. I just couldn't get away from Stanford, so Karyn chose the house, negotiated with the real-estate agents, signed the papers. And while I set up the transplant program, she moved us in, redecorated the place, created the home where my children played in the airy, spacious rooms, on the large terraced grounds, and in the woodsy backyard, and where once or twice a week I managed to drop by for a visit.

I didn't realize I had slept until the hypnotic drone of the powerful jet engines changed abruptly and I heard Rusty and Nancy beginning to stir.

The lights of the city came into focus atop buildings and along deserted streets. Soon we were streaking over the blacktop of the runway, hearing the scream of rubber below. We taxied for about five minutes before we pulled up to the waiting helicopter, its rotors already turning.

As the doors to the jet opened, Rusty leaned forward and shouted to the pilot over the roar of the engines. "We've got to do better with the taxiing time on the way back. Don't pick us up here. Get ready for takeoff, wait for us at the end of the runway. The helicopter can drop us there." He paused, looked at the pilot, and went on. "I'll call you from the hospital, let you know exactly when we will get back. Once we get the heart, every second counts."

Rusty smiled when the pilot nodded, and we dived out into the steamy Florida air.

We ducked under the whomp, whomp, whomp of the helicopter blades and lifted off. Tampa, the little toy town in the darkness below, was slumbering, but when we reached the hospital, the pilot nudged my arm, pointing to the parking lot. There sat a fire truck and two ambulances parked in a triangle, their lights flashing red and yellow. The piercing headlights from all three were trained on a central area they wanted us to use as a landing pad.

15

The pilot was laughing at all the fuss. There was hardly a car in the hospital's lot, and he could have set down virtually anywhere. As we got closer, we could see a group of people, firemen included, watching the night sky for our arrival.

"Look at 'em," Rusty said. "They've gone to a lot of trouble."

We both were smiling, both thinking the same thing. I had been worrying all the way from the airport about being out of touch with the hospital for over an hour and a half, wondering if the donor was still stable, if any problems had come up, if they could handle them, if they'd called Walter with new information. I could tell Rusty had worried, too. Given the reception, the care they seemed to have taken, we both relaxed a bit.

"My dad loves little hospitals like this," I said, as we walked over to meet the crowd. "That's one of the biggest kicks he gets out of Hospital Corporation of America. Going around to the little community hospitals they own. Talking to the administrators, touring the facilities, praising the nurses, swapping stories with the doctors.

" 'They are people places,' he says."

3

While our Lear was making its breathtaking trip, Jim Hayes had been roaring along at a mere seventy or so miles an hour up Interstate 40 from Knoxville. For most heart-transplant patients, the kind of trip Jim was making tonight would be the longest of their lives. But he had made the trip before.

He knew what lay in store for him: the long stay in the hospital after the operation; the first, almost inevitable episode of rejection when his body's immune system would begin to attack his new heart as an alien threat; the long search for the right combination of drugs to hold the immune system in check, drugs with names now so familiar to him that it was hard to remember when they sounded odd, exotic, even a little frightening: azathioprine, prednisone, cyclosporine, OKT3. There would be frequent biopsies, when his doctors would run a tiny pair of tweezers down a tube stuck in a vein of his neck and clip off five little pieces of his heart muscle to study and analyze; weeks of physical therapy, slowly bringing his new heart and his atrophied leg and arm muscles up to snuff and into harmony with one another; and finally the lifelong regimen of watching what he ate, taking a dozen different medicines daily at just the right time, and paying close, careful attention to every sneeze and sniffle, each cut or sore that appeared on his body, the slightest variation in his temperature.

Jim knew that it took a certain kind of person to be a good heart-transplant recipient. He was that kind of person. He had been at it almost as long as anyone alive. When he got his first transplant, they hadn't even discovered cyclosporine. Even his own doctors thought at the time that he had only an even chance of being alive five years later. In fact, it was hard for him to

17

remember back to a time when he didn't have someone else's heart.

He could remember his pretransplant army days in Germany, the days when his father was still alive. He remembered how he had so disappointed the man. For years, he hid the fact that he had a daughter born out of wedlock from his father. He had not wanted to marry her mother, knowing that he did not love the woman. In the army, a world away from the confusion back home, he remembered feeling sure of himself, certain that no God existed, that a man was only what he made of himself. Everything would work out.

Back then, he thought of himself as healthy and normal and a pretty good sort of guy; now *that* life seemed to belong to someone else, *that* life seemed to him the sick one. Not until the day he woke up and found he couldn't walk across a room without help, not until he learned he had an incurable heart disease, not until he understood he might die very soon indeed did he begin to think he had been wasting his life.

His faith in God had come back early, the minute in fact that someone had told him he was going to die, but his faith in life—that took longer. The transplant—the risks involved, its experimental nature, the long, agonizing wait for a donor—taught him to value life, each precious moment of it, but it did not teach him how to live. He had tried to do the right things, to face up to his father and tell him the truth about his child, to marry the mother and provide a decent home. But it had turned out badly. His father died while Jim was waiting for his new heart. His wife began drinking heavily, and for a long time he blamed himself and the pressure of his stringent postoperative course.

He felt guilty about everything. Guilty that he wasn't working, that his wife was so miserable, that someone had to die in order for him to live. When it became clear that his wife was an alcoholic, he tried to stick with her but couldn't. He even botched the divorce, remarrying on the rebound. The second marriage lasted barely a year.

Although he didn't know it at the time, the road back started in a health club in California shortly after his transplant. A young woman who worked at the club walked up to him one day and said, "You're Jim Hayes, right? You have my brother's heart." She explained that her teenage brother had been killed in a car accident and that she had gotten Jim's name from a nurse she knew at the Stanford hospital.

They met once a week, and she told him about her brother and her family. She had told her folks that she had met Jim, and they wanted to know all about him. They didn't want to see him, they didn't think they could face that, but they did want him to know that they were pleased with how well he was doing.

Jim stayed in touch with the woman over the years and saw her on each of his annual visits. When he made his bike trip across the country on the fifth anniversary of his transplant, her parents asked to meet him.

The bike trip marked the turning point for him. From the moment he told the doctors what he planned, the will to live a better life had begun to grow in him; when he actually made the trip, that will became indomitable. He and his donor's parents grew very close. They saw in him their son's life redeemed from tragedy. He felt that by going on, by making it day to day, he was fulfilling the promise of their son's existence.

He had found a purpose, and slowly he overcame his guilt. He got out of his second marriage. He focused his energy on caring for his daughter. He tried to be the man his father had been. By the time he met Shirley, everything was ready to fall into place. Together they made a real marriage, and she gave him a son. She sat by his side now as he sped down the highway toward what for almost anybody else would be a terrifying event. For him it seemed nearly normal.

He had faith, love, a desire to live, and the knowledge that life was a gift, not an inalienable right.

It had served him well when he learned that his "new" heart was failing.

When the team at Stanford told Jim that he would need a third heart, he worried most about the parents whose dead son had been the donor for his first operation. He was going to clip the one thread that still connected them to their boy. He was afraid to lose them, afraid to lose the bond that had brought meaning to his life. They reassured him, encouraging him to move as quickly as possible. If their son's gift truly had meaning, it came from giving Jim a second chance. What good was that now if he died?

One might suspect that Jim would fear another wait, the unnecessary torture that all transplant patients go through: hoping for holiday weekends when accidental deaths are more common and hating themselves for it; comparing themselves to other transplant recipients they met in the course of diagnosis and intermediary treatment; worrying about the fairness of the computerized procurement system, the honesty of other surgeons, and the good intentions of their own. More than most, Jim knew the odds were against him. But he had beaten the odds for a long time. And he had Shirley.

The Stanford doctors told Jim that a new transplant program was starting up at Vanderbilt and that one of their own would be in charge of it. He could get the same care he was used to without traveling a thousand miles and living in overpriced hotels or apartments.

As one of the longest-living heart-transplant recipients, he knew what to look for in a program. He had come to Vanderbilt earlier for a routine cardiac biopsy, which had not gone well. Afterward, he headed straight back to the West Coast. He told the Stanford nurses that he'd received unsatisfactory care at Vanderbilt. They urged him to meet with me and give it another try. He fought their advice, insisting that he knew the difference between good care and the kind of shoddy treatment he had received in Nashville. Eventually he relented, and almost a year ago he and Shirley had walked warily into my office.

Later he would tell me that he knew within minutes that I was the guy for him. I reminded him, he told me, of Dr. Bill Baumgartner, a mild-mannered, warm, and affable Kentuckian who had done Jim's first transplant. Jim adored him. I knew that what Jim appreciated was the Stanford style of care created by pioneer transplant surgeon Norman Shumway. He and the rather atypical cardiac surgeons he had attracted to his program had developed a low-key but highly disciplined approach to transplantation practiced at Stanford. It was an approach I very much believed in, and Jim personified for me how well it worked.

Also, I had no difficulty sensing the real fighter in Jim Hayes. It was this tenacious spirit on which I now counted—in addition to the new heart I had yet to see and my abilities as a surgeon—to get us both through the long night ahead. And the years that followed.

He was much on my mind as our little party met the group welcoming us to the Florida hospital. By now, Jim and Shirley should have pulled into the parking garage across from Vanderbilt's main building, locked up, and trekked through the crisp Nashville night, across the deserted streets, and into the hospital. As the hospital administrator, flashlight in hand, led us into his modern three-story facility, I looked anxiously for a telephone to call Walter.

"It's a big night for us," the administrator said. "We've never done a heart before, and it's all anybody round here can talk about."

We headed down a long hallway that began to fill up with nurses and technicians and others stepping out of doorways to view the intruders. They watched us march along behind their boss, carrying our little red and white cooler, so commonplace yet so vital to the whole process. We changed into fresh scrubs. As Rusty and Nancy walked off in their blues to check out the operating room, I broke away and made my call.

Jim Hayes had indeed already arrived, and surgical resident Tom Wareing had taken him directly to his room on Seven North.

"Jan's been up there already," Walter said. "Gave him a quick once-over and says his condition is good. Wareing took a look at his chart, checked him out for any infections. Lab tests are back, including blood count and bleeding studies. I looked at his chest x-ray, and it's clear. Seems weird not to be ordering a bunch of immunosuppressants."

"I know," I said. Jim was our first retransplant. He was already on a full immunosuppressive regimen. "All sounds good. I'll call you back in approximately forty-five minutes, soon as I open the chest and get a look at the thing. Better not cut skin there until I'm sure it looks as good as we think." We didn't want to cut open Jim's chest if the heart here in Florida wasn't suitable.

Briefly, I thought how Jim had sounded calmer than I felt when he called me from the road. I had seen press clippings of his bike trip and watched a videotape he had given me of "That's Incredible!"—an old television show that had covered his trip. They had made something of a circus out of it, much to Jim's irritation. Biking across the country, pedaling against the vicious Kansas winds, racing through the Rockies just ahead of a snowstorm—the guy's going to be just fine, I said to myself.

Rusty was standing outside the OR telling Nancy about our run to Boston a few weeks back. The cool reception we had gotten. Waiting four hours for them to free up an operating room. No doubt about it, some places simply resented transplant teams with their strange demands that disrupted the normal hospital routines. Operating schedules had to be changed, scrub nurses called in after hours. I could understand the feeling, but I didn't have much sympathy. The Jim Hayeses of the world were simply too real for me.

"Kidney team's working on the donor now," Rusty said as I pulled on a surgical mask. "Been here about an hour. Bone people are in line, waiting their turn."

"I guess I'd better get in there, take a look."

I sounded calm, level, in control, despite the quick flash of irritation I felt at the other teams for jumping the gun, for starting their work before we arrived. I thought about the folks up in Boston, and I smiled behind my mask. So many surgeons from so many different places—it was amazing how smoothly it all worked.

4

The first heart I ever saw was a dog's.

During my second year at Harvard Medical School, the other students and I performed surgery on animals as part of Dr. Cliff Barger's physiology class. It was the highlight of the second year of medical school because we actually saw for the first time the very organs, live and functioning, that until then had been mere pictures and text in our books, just subjects for us to agonizingly memorize.

As part of our physiology class, we had removed a dog's spleen. At the end of the operation, we sacrificed the animal by cutting out its heart. One of the students handed the heart to me. As it lay in my palm, it continued to beat for a minute or so. To me it seemed an eternity: I was hooked.

As my associates walked away from the table to review the laboratory data, I could not put the heart down. I stared at it cradled in my hand, spellbound. Amazed that it could still beat outside the body, I took a scalpel and cut through the heart's thick, muscled wall, then stood gawking at the delicate valve leaflets, so impossibly thin that I could see right through them. They were suspended from the wall by narrow, glistening, sculptured cords. Just a simple pump, I thought. But in contrast to its straightforward function, its internal structure seemed so complex, so intricate.

By the time I left the lab that day, I knew I would devote my career to the study of this miraculous organ. Though my fascination was scientific, medical, it was more as well. Like most of us, I had a sentimental attachment to the heart and its many mystical associations. As a hollow, muscular organ that circulates blood through the body, a heart is not much different from a liver, a pancreas, the lungs—all vital anatomical parts we cannot live without. But most of us *feel* the heart working in ways that we believe are beyond physiology. Our hearts race, or skip a beat, or break, we say, and we are gripped by fear, heavy with sadness, filled with joy, lost in love. From remote time, mankind has considered the heart the sanctuary of our emotions.

I would come to know surgeons who thought of the heart in strictly anatomical terms, who viewed its functions as a purely technical matter. But I had fallen under a spell that afternoon in Dr. Barger's class, and I never lost my feeling of awe. It was one of the major reasons I was in this business, the secret behind my standing outside an operating room in Florida, glancing with some anxiety through a donor's chart, double-checking the official pronouncement of brain death, the family consent form, the patient's blood type, hoping to find some magic sign hidden in the paperwork that said this heart will be strong, this heart will be healthy, this heart will be good.

I was relieved to see from the charts that the donor's blood pressure had not dropped drastically at any point since the accident, as it sometimes does when the brain herniates. I was pleased that he had been given only moderate doses of dopamine and had been kept on adequate fluids. The electrocardiogram looked good, heart rate normal, no suggestion of damage to the muscle. The chest x-ray was clear, the lungs had not collapsed or developed any pneumonia. I looked at Rusty.

"We were joking about little hospitals," I said. "But we're probably better off here than we are in some place like that huge one in Boston. They don't get so many trauma cases at once. If they just knew the basics of donor management."

"Yeah," Rusty laughed. "And if they got somebody like me yelling at 'em constantly."

"Right. But I feel good about this. I was getting worried because I don't like people going in there and working away before I get here to manage the heart. But this looks good."

24

That was when I glanced through the small glass pane in the operating room door.

The anesthesiologist was perched on a stool reading *Time* magazine. Next to him was the draped head of the donor. My eyes shot up to the cardiac monitor bolted to the ceiling. He hadn't even placed an arterial line in the body to monitor the blood pressure.

Rusty saw it too. I slung down the file, pushed open the door. Behind me, Rusty called, "Dr. Frist!"

The anesthesiologist looked up as I came over. He may not have seen the anger in my eyes, but I doubt it.

"You put in an arterial line?"

"No," he said. "I didn't think it seemed indicated."

As he answered, I looked at all the lines stretching up from underneath the drapes. No central venous line, which we normally thread down a blood vessel into the heart to monitor how well a patient is hydrated. Only one small volume line. Without larger lines, there was no way the anesthesiologist could pump fluids, including blood, quickly into the patient should the blood pressure drop or the donor start to lose blood unexpectedly.

"How about a central venous line?"

"No," he said.

"Volume lines?" I snapped.

He shrugged. "Just the one," he said, nodding his head toward a tube that looked even smaller than when I first glanced at it.

"Could we step over here for a minute?" I said, moving away from the operating table and out of earshot of the others.

He looked at me, looked at the surgeons around the table already operating, looked at the nurse assisting them. It was on the tip of my tongue to say, Not much you could do if anything happened, is there? But I held back. Calm, I thought. Calm.

"Hey—," he said.

"No, No," I said. "I understand. They called you in the middle of the night to get out of bed to come into the hospital to take care of a brain-dead patient. Not exactly what you'd call a challenging, exciting night in the operating room."

"I do my job," he said.

"Not tonight you didn't. I've got a patient waiting for a heart up there in Nashville, a man who will die if I don't give him the heart there."

"He'll get it."

"Will he? If your patient's blood pressure begins to drop, how are you going to know what caused it without a central line? How are you going to know how to respond? You can't. Let's just suppose those fellows over there—no matter how good they are— accidentally cause a little bleeding while they're taking out the kidneys? His blood pressure drops, the heart arrests, develops arrhythmias, whatever. How are you going to pump blood, flu-ids, all of that fast enough while we handle the emergency? You can't. We lose the heart. My patient in Nashville dies."

"I—" ·

"Same thing with the kidneys. Something happens to them, two of their patients go back on dialysis, at best to wait months or years for another chance. That body there—it means two other people will get to see because they've got new corneas, others will get bone grafts. That brain-dead body over there may seem worth-less in your eyes, but it will directly affect the lives of maybe fifteen other people—and so could your goofing off."

He started to say something else, but I cut him short again. "This is no place to be bored or indifferent, *Doctor*. It's too late to put in the lines we need to do this thing right, but at least get rid of the magazine. You are a doctor. Act like one."

He nodded, then went back to his job. The magazine stayed out of sight, and I felt a little better. At least I was no longer angry. I introduced myself to the two surgeons. They told me their names, looking up from the task at hand just long enough for a nod.

"Where you from?" I asked.

"Miami," the taller one answered.

"How long you think you'll be?"

"Forty-five minutes, if that."

26

"I'll go ahead and scrub up so I can take a look at the heart, if that's okay with you. But I'll wait till you've done your dissection to take it out."

They both nodded. They wouldn't remove the kidneys until I had the heart. The sequence follows the best physiological progression, not the order of arrival. First the heart, then the liver and kidneys, then corneas, bone, and other tissue. They had been doing preparatory work: it takes an hour or so to free up the kidneys, two to isolate the liver, but only thirty minutes or so to open up the chest and inspect and prepare the heart.

I glanced at the ECG monitor above the donor's head, looked at the chest x-ray film posted on a fluorescent viewing screen in the corner, checked the anesthesiologist's records. The ECG tracing was normal and so was the heart silhouette on x-ray, but the flow sheet showed that the donor's blood pressure had been falling slowly over the past thirty minutes. Just as I had warned the anesthesiologist, there was no way to understand why it was dropping without a central line. Something was wrong. I had to get a look at the heart quickly.

"His blood pressure's falling," I said. "Step up the dopamine and give him as much crystalloid fluid as possible. I'll be right back." I left to scrub.

Rusty had been standing off to the side with the retractor and other surgical equipment we'd brought. He handed it to the nurse and joined me at the scrub sink outside the OR. The anesthesiologist's attitude still bothered me, but I fought the impulse to complain to Rusty. Once was enough. I had to get the chest open.

Eight minutes later the timer above the sink went off, and I rinsed the soap from my hands. A nurse came through the OR door.

"You a seven-and-a-half glove?"

"Right."

I followed her back into the OR, dripping arms held chest high, took the towel from the scrub nurse, dried my hands, and stepped into the sterile green gown as she tore open a packet of gloves. I met her eyes above her mask as she snapped the gloves in place. In an operating room, you talk with your eyes about

27

anything that doesn't have to do with the surgery. Her eyes said, Makes me nervous, all you strangers.

"Don't worry," I said. "I'll explain everything you need to know, step by step, as we go along. Let's start with the equipment."

When I mentioned the electric sternal saw that I would need to cut through the breastbone, her eyes said, Oh, God.

"What's wrong?"

"Don't have one," she said.

"You don't have an electric saw? Do you have a sternal knife?"

"No, I'm really sorry."

"Don't worry," I said. "Some heavy scissors will do fine." I thought to myself, At least it'll be a challenge.

And her eyes were smiling.

The donor's blood pressure was responding nicely to the fluid push, a sign that the heart was working well.

I took my place to the donor's right, adjacent to his chest and directly across from the scrub nurse. One kidney surgeon stood to my right, the other across the table. Another surgical assistant was next to him, holding an abdominal-wall retractor. Scalpel in hand, I cut down the center of the chest. Then I went after the thick, hard breastbone with a pair of heavy scissors, a first for me. It felt strange not to hear the searing buzz sound or smell the acrid scent of the electric saw. I thought how much easier all this would have been back at Vanderbilt.

My adrenalin began pumping as I got ready to open the pericardial sac that holds the heart. This is it, I thought. One more move, and I'll know. I did not allow myself to think that what I found in the next instant might mean the difference between life and death for Jim Hayes, but I could feel my own heart beating faster as I slit open the sac.

The heart below me was pumping away, beating rhythmically and vigorously.

It's perfect, I thought. Just perfect.

28

5

I took hold of the young heart. I had to make sure it really was as perfect as it looked.

Blood flows back continuously into the heart through the veins, only to be shot out from the pulsating organ into the thicker vessels called arteries, carrying oxygen and nutrients to all parts of the body. The heart, little larger than one's fist, is divided in half by a muscular membrane, the septum. Each half in turn has a thin-walled receiving chamber called the atrium and a more muscular ejecting chamber called the ventricle. The blood pours into and out of the ventricles through valves, the tricuspid and pulmonary valves in the right ventricle, the mitral and aortic valves in the left. Each and every day, the heart pumps 2,000 gallons of blood, expanding and contracting over 100,000 times. A tireless organ.

Smoking, high blood pressure, birth defects, and elevated blood cholesterol can all damage the arteries, the valve leaflets, and the muscular chambers and can destroy the heart's ability to pump blood through the body. My job now was to look for signs of such damage. I stroked, or palpated, the heart to get a sense of its strength. I felt the atrium in each half, seeking a "thrill," a little flutter, like water running rapidly through a pipe, that meant a heart valve was not functioning properly. It would sound like a murmur through a stethoscope. Next, I ran my finger gently down the course of each of the three major coronary arteries. These vessels lie on the surface of the heart and feed the indefatigably beating muscle oxygen and nutrients. I was looking for plaque, or the hardening of the arteries that would signify coronary-artery disease.

There was no thrill. The arteries were soft and smooth. The

heart was free of disease, ideal. Relieved, I broke scrub, took off my gown.

"One of you fellows let me know as soon as you're finished," I said to the kidney surgeons, and I left to call Walter.

People still milled around in the hall outside the OR. As I walked to the phone, I heard them talking to newcomers: Doing a heart. Right now. In there. That's him, down there, on the phone. The guy that just walked by. Nashville. I caught Walter on his beeper, but he was already in the office.

"Heart looks fine," I said. "But we'd better push back our estimated time of arrival in Nashville by thirty-five minutes. These kidney surgeons are pretty green. How's it going at your end?"

"Good. Good. When should we take Jim to OR?"

"Let's go ahead, get him in there, get his lines in, and put him to sleep in exactly one hour." As Walter concurred and said his good-byes, I wrote the agreed-upon time down on the pant leg of my scrub suit. On the way to the doctors' lounge, where the Florida folks had set up coffee and donuts, I stopped by the OR again. The donor's blood pressure had dropped again as the kidney surgeons continued their abdominal dissection, exposing the intestines to air and allowing fluids to evaporate. I told the anesthesiologist to give more fluid, then left. I grabbed a chocolate donut, two cups of coffee, and a catnap.

He must have called my name. There he was, shaking me by the shoulder. It seemed very strange that he wasn't saying anything. Just shaking me.

"Rusty?" I said.

"The boys from Miami say ten minutes."

I scrubbed. Rusty filled the Igloo cooler with ice. Nancy stood there with the scrub nurse. Both Nancy and Rusty had been fully trained as nurses, and they had been through this before, but it didn't hurt for them to hear me explain to the uninitiated scrub nurse precisely what I would be doing and what I wanted everyone to do.

"First, I'll inject a solution into the heart to make it stop suddenly. Then I'll pour buckets of ice-cold saline onto the heart to try to get it as cold as possible. I'll need five liters of real cold stuff—either Ringer's lactate or normal saline—on your table as soon as we start. Nancy, you show her how to line up the buckets of saline so we can move quickly." I looked at the nurse. "It's very, very important that I get the real cold stuff as soon as I ask for it. No delays.

"It won't take more than a couple of minutes to excise the heart. The instant it's cut free, we start the countdown for isch-emic time—when there's no blood flowing to the heart. From then on, every second counts. I'll put the heart in that sterile plastic bowl and rinse it thoroughly to get rid of the old blood. Next, I'll stick it in the two plastic bags, then into the plastic container, then into the cooler. At that moment, we're out of here.

"Nancy will make sure everything we brought is ready to go." I turned to her, nodding my head. "Don't let me forget the retractor. Also, have someone tell the helicopter pilot we're now precisely five minutes from takeoff. Rusty, call Walter now and let him know our exact timing. Tell him we'll be back on the jet, ready to take off, in twenty-two minutes and to go ahead and put Jim to sleep. Okay, let's do it."

The other surgeons stepped back. Every eye in the room focused on the heart. The surgery went smoothly. I worked fast, and the OR team picked up the tempo. Two minutes later, I lifted the now limp heart out of the donor's chest and cupped it gently in both my hands as I turned to walk over to the instrument table. Hearts are slippery, but you don't want to hold them too tightly. I always feared that I would drop one. I placed it quickly but carefully into the saline-filled plastic basin.

I noticed how quiet it was. A hush had fallen over the room.

I wasn't the only one who held the heart in awe, and I had seen this before, even with the most experienced operating-room staffs. I held the symbolic center of life in my hands. Yesterday it had fueled a man's normal activities. A few minutes ago we'd all seen it beating strong and sure, the way it had beaten some billion times before. Now it lay isolated and inert in my hands.

I rinsed the heart in the cold saline and slipped it into the large plastic bag Rusty held open. We poured more real cold stuff into the bag, twisted it shut, and tied it with an ordinary super-market twist tie. Then the second bag. Then the plastic container, its lid snapped closed. Finally I buried it all deep in the ice of the Igloo picnic chest.

Rusty was gone. I jumped out of my gown, popped off my gloves, said my thank-yous to the OR staff, and took off after him. Nancy brought up the rear, toting our equipment in a blue canvas gym bag. A gray dawn was fighting its way through drizzling rain as we dashed for the helicopter, revved and ready to go. A crowd of twenty or so had followed us on our march down the long hospital corridors. When we lifted off, they stood on the wet asphalt, in the rain, waving good-bye.

The pilot couldn't see a thing. He kept us low, at 300 feet, all the way to the airport. Rusty sat there with the Igloo cooler held tight in his hands as we skimmed the treetops and skirted electrical wires and swept over the looming tops of tall buildings. I imag-ined the first horrible snap of impact, envisioned the circling plunge toward earth, and in my mind saw Rusty calmly clutching the cooler all the way down.

I could hear the radio. Air traffic control told us to hold. Another aircraft was making an approach, an instrument landing. I knew they might make us hold a pattern for five minutes or more. I picked up the microphone, called the controller.

"Approach, this is LifeFlight, Four Kilo Bravo. We have a live organ aboard. Request immediate clearance to the run-up area, runway fifteen."

Something worked. Probably the urgency in my voice. He cleared us immediately. I could see our Lear in position at the end of the runway, poised for takeoff. A blink later we were climbing fast through the heavy haze toward the dark clouds above. Abruptly, we were in another world. At 10,000 feet, popping through the rain clouds, the sky was a clear cornflower blue.

We climbed to 20,000 feet and leveled off. I looked at Rusty. At the cooler. At the heart, sleeping on ice, thousands and thousands of its cells dying every minute it was out of the body, every second it failed to pump.

Even to me it all seemed a bit bizarre, this flying around in the middle of the night with a heart in a cooler. If someone had told Dad fifty years ago when he began practicing medicine what I would be doing that night, he would have laughed and shook his head in disbelief, dismissing it all as pure science fiction.

"Pilot has called Nashville with our ETA," Rusty said. "Still want to take the ambulance to Vandy, or should we get the chopper?"

"No, I don't think so." A helicopter wouldn't make much difference in the few miles we had to go between the airport and Vanderbilt, but it would cost twenty times more. "The ambulance will be just as fast this time of morning. We'll miss rush hour, don't you think?"

"We should," Rusty said.

I looked at my watch, checking the time against the estimate I had scribbled on my pant leg. Two minutes off. Not bad. It was six in the morning.

"Jet lands on time, the ambulance doesn't have a flat, we don't get in a wreck, we'll make it with time to spare," Rusty said.

"Lotta ifs in this business," I laughed, able to relax some since there was nothing I could do in flight. It's a good thing I don't fly my own plane on these runs. "One time at Stanford we sent our team to a small town. Someplace in Oregon. Middle of the night. On the way back, they take off and one of the jet engines sucks up a bird. The airport was so small there wasn't even a telephone. They had no way to tell us back at Stanford that they couldn't get off the ground. Last we heard, they had the heart on ice and were headed out the door of the hospital. We assumed everything was on schedule. The grounded pilots finally make radio contact with a Delta plane flying by. They contacted a Delta reservations clerk in Chicago. She called me in the OR back at Stanford, right before I made the skin incision. I said, OK, but I kept asking myself how a Delta reservations clerk in Chicago knew that our donor heart in Oregon was being delayed."

"The heart get there in time?"

"Barely," I said. "They finally found another charter jet in an airport a hundred miles down the road. The ischemic time was over four hours, but the recipient ultimately did well. A close call. That's all we talked about at Stanford for weeks.

"I know a couple of times people have grabbed the wrong coolers getting off the plane," I went on. "Pilots use these Igloos all the time. For juice, soft drinks. They all look alike. Just think about it. You get back to the operating room, open up the Igloo, and pull out a Pepsi instead of the heart."

We all three laughed.

"True story," I said.

"Yeah," Rusty said, looking at the cooler. "You hear about stuff like that."

Davidson County stretched out below us in the bright early morning light, its farms and lakes and pastures and hills and valleys a patchwork quilt of colors. We packed up, Rusty never letting go of the cooler for long, even when he put it on the seat next to him. Minutes later, siren screaming, we braced ourselves for the ambulance ride. But for some perverse reason the young driver seemed reluctant to take full advantage of his right of way. He weaved in and out of traffic at forty miles an hour when he should have done sixty, and he crept along the interstate at sixty when he should have topped eighty.

The ride was not shaping up to be the harrowing experience I both expected and desired. I looked at my watch. Rusty looked at his watch. Nancy looked at her watch. What ought to have taken twelve minutes was stretching into twenty. Rusty did not say to me *Should have taken the copter.*

At last we pulled into Vanderbilt's emergency entrance. As we hopped out, we could see the receptionist on the phone to Walter in the OR. It was his signal to put Jim on bypass and start cutting out his sick heart. We skipped the elevator. Hospital

34

elevators are notoriously slow. Sometimes they fail. Who wants to get caught between floors with a heart that's deteriorating by the second? We took the stairs to the third floor, two at a time. I changed one last time into fresh scrubs. Nancy and Rusty went on ahead with the cooler.

When you're standing there in the OR ready to take out somebody's heart, you hold your breath till your associate actually walks into the room, cooler in hand. We don't do anything irreversible to the recipient until the heart hits the hospital, but those last few minutes before it reaches the operating room can be awfully tense.

"Hey," Walter said in his usual understated way as I walked into the OR. "You made it!"

"Good run," I said. "How about you?"

"We're ready when you are."

I looked at the monitor in the corner and watched Jim's ECG flatten. Having placed him on total heart-lung bypass, Walter was snipping out the diseased heart that had nevertheless served Jim well for more than a decade.

"Just let me go over to that cooler," I said, "and get me a Pepsi."

When they had come for him this time, Jim was awake and alert. He had spent part of the night talking excitedly to Jan Muirhead, and Dr. Merrill had come up just before they wheeled him out. Dr. Merrill was his usual casual, easygoing self, and Jim figured he was trying to calm him down. Later Jim said he felt like telling Walter, "Hey, it's OK, Doc. I know what's going on. I've been here before."

As they rolled down the corridor, Jim watched the numbers of the plastic plaques next to the operating room doors, playing a game with himself, trying to guess his lucky number. OR 5—no. OR 6—no. OR 7—no. They turned at OR 8. Inside, Dr. Merrill and Jan and a number of nurses and surgical residents puttered about, all wearing masks, all talking in the quiet tones Jim had come to associate with surgery.

35

The room was supermarket bright and totally without character—pictureless beige walls, stainless-steel tables draped in pale blue-green, an assortment of odd-looking instruments carefully laid out like alien tableware, so clean and hushed that normal sounds and street dress seemed not just out of place, but sinful. There was a television set hanging from the ceiling in one corner and those weird machines—with their computer-blue and gray casings, their flickering screens, their gauges—stacked behind him, standing by either side, off in corners.

On the machines closest to him, he could read the labels: OHMEDA Modulus II Anesthesia System, IMED 960 Volumetric Infusion Pump, CHEMETRON Medical Division System for Anesthetic and Respiratory Analysis, OHMEDA 5420 Volume Monitor, 5210 CO_2 Monitor, OHMEDA 7000 Ventilator. They were numbered, in no particular order, with bright red stick-on labels—3, 12, 31, 38—and their screens and gauges said things like Air, Helium, Nitrous Oxide, Oxygen, Pipeline, Cylinder. All of it had something to do with him, all this science and equipment, all these people, the words, the sounds, all wired to his body now, with the IV the anesthesiologist was putting in his arm, all intent on him. The money, the training, the twists of fate, all helping him live a little longer. He couldn't disappoint them, he had to make it.

He had been surprised that so far they had given him no medication. Last time, he had started taking the immunosuppressive medicines as soon as he had arrived at the hospital. The painful shots in his thighs. But of course they didn't have to this time. He lived on the stuff, day in and day out. Look at the clock. Time to take more medicine. Sun's up. Time to swallow pills. You hungry? Take a dose.

He realized now that something was seeping into his veins . . . from the machines . . . liquid in clear plastic bags hanging on a pole over his head . . . dripping . . . he could see but he couldn't hear . . . bright, blinding spotlights . . . now he could hear the anesthesiologist's soft voice, talking, talking, talking. . . . "Think of a sweet dream, Jim," the voice whispered. . . . "See you in a minute or two," it said. . . . And another whisper, "In the recovery room."

Once Jim had been put to sleep with intravenous medication, the anesthesiologist took a long tube attached to a ventilator and pushed its free end into Jim's mouth, down between his vocal cords, and into his windpipe. During the operation the ventilator would blow air rhythmically down this endotracheal tube, breathing for him. Next, Tom Wareing, the chief surgical resident I'd called earlier, poked a catheter into the artery in Jim's left wrist. With this small arterial line we could accurately monitor his blood pressure, moment by moment. Tom stuck another catheter into a vein high on Jim's chest; through this tube we could give him medicines and measure his intravascular volume. Tom also ran a small tube up Jim's penis to drain his bladder so we could follow his urine output. Then Tom prepped Jim, shaving off his body hair, swabbing him down with soap and water, and painting him with two coats of iodine. Finally Jim was draped, his entire body covered with sterile sheets except for a strip of exposed chest and upper abdomen.

This area, dull orange from the iodine, covered with tightly drawn clear plastic, was all the surgeons would see of Jim Hayes when they walked into the operating room. Called the surgical field, it was both clean and intentionally dehumanized, an area on which surgeons could focus all their attention and energy without being overly worried about infection or distracted by the fact that they actually knew this man, talked to him, liked him, even admired him. The OR has little room for germs or personalities.

If Jim had been just another transplant patient, Walter would have made an incision from Jim's lower neck down the center of his chest to the upper abdomen, cutting clear through the skin and fat and muscle till he reached his breastbone, or sternum. Then—God willing, using a small electric saw—he would cut the sternum down the middle. But Jim already had a fine, well-healed scar from just such an incision made eleven years earlier at Stanford by Drs. Shumway and Baumgartner. As a result, there was a mass of dense scar tissue, or adhesions, between the back side of Jim's breastbone and his heart. Walter had to divide the scar carefully, making sure not to injure the heart.

Once the incision was made, Walter and Tom pried the chest open with a heavy chest spreader, pulling from either side like men in a modified tug of war. Walter checked out the heart. There would be no pericardial sac around this heart the way there had been on the donor. This heart was connected only to Jim's major blood vessels, not to his nerves. He could have had a massive heart attack and never known it, since without nerves he would have felt no pain. Jim's heart did not even look much like those we usually removed. Most of these hearts, suffering from a condition called dilated cardiomyopathy, were two or three times the size of a normal heart—big, flabby, swollen sacs that barely seemed to beat.

Jim's was normal size, but the coronary arteries were rock hard.

Walter went back to work freeing the heart from the surrounding scar tissue. He put one suture into the ascending aorta, the big blood vessel responsible for carrying blood from the heart to the rest of the body. Then he placed two sutures in the right atrium. In a moment he would insert tubes, called cannulas, through these three purse-string sutures in order to connect Jim to the heart-lung bypass machine. First he had to shoot a drug called heparin directly into the heart to keep Jim's blood from clotting as it passed through the oxygenator and bypass machine.

That done, Jim went on bypass. The tubes shunted Jim's blood away from his heart and ran it into a squat, mobile metal cabinet on the floor behind Walter. On one side of the cardiopulmonary bypass machine was a row of transparent canisters with whirling blades, looking a little like high-tech versions of those old ice-cream makers. As Jim's veins fed blood into the canisters, the machine gave it oxygen and then pumped the enriched blood out again, back into Jim's ascending aorta.

On the opposite side of the bypass machine, a young technician called a perfusionist watched a series of calibrated gauges labelled Arterial Vent, Cardiac Sucker, and Remote Temperatures, piloting the machine and making sure that Jim's blood was circulating as it should. The anesthesiologist too was checking a series of gauges and screens, tracing Jim's heart rate, his blood pressure, the central venous pressure, how much carbon dioxide Jim exhaled, how much oxygen his lungs took in. From time to time, when one of the two noticed something amiss, they would say in what might appear a casual, off-hand observation, "Pressure's getting low," or, "Flow's fallen off."

But the casualness was deceptive, a professional tone we all cultivated. Walter would understand the seriousness of the statement; his eyes would flicker up to the television monitor suspended in the corner, where he could see Jim's blood pressure for himself; he would keep working, trying to correct the problem immediately.

But none of that happened as Jim went on bypass and Walter began to cut out his heart. Because it was Jim's second transplant, the whole process took longer than normal, and Walter was just making the final cut to remove the heart when I stepped into my appointed place on the left, across from him. Behind him, the perfusionist sat on a low stool in front of the bypass machine. Tom Wareing stood to my left, the scrub nurse next to him. The anesthesiologist held vigil at Jim's head, to my right. I made a quick check of the monitor hanging from the ceiling and glanced over the entire crew with something like relief.

It felt good to be back at Vanderbilt among familiar faces, with people I knew and trusted and could relax with. One operating room looks much like another, but the atmosphere is always different. I liked mine calm, efficient, congenial, the way Dr. Shumway's was at Stanford. During medical school at Harvard and as a resident in Boston, I'd seen too many arrogant, demanding, insensitive surgeons create a tense, uptight atmosphere, where everyone on the team walked around on eggshells worrying more about the temperament of the surgeon than the welfare of the patient. Efficiency, perfection, and order were musts, but throwing instruments and humiliating others never made much sense to me.

Then Walter handed me Jim's still-beating heart, and I dropped it into a metal pan on the stand at the foot of the operating table. On the same stand, not far away, lay the new heart in a sterile basin. I was running my finger along the old heart's left anterior descending coronary artery when Walter came around the end to inspect it as well.

"Try to squeeze that artery. It's a rock," I said.

"It's a miracle any blood got through there at all," Walter responded.

Jim Atkinson walked into the room.

"Hear you got a sick one for me," he said.

Atkinson is our cardiac pathologist. Each time we do a transplant, he shows up day or night to take the old heart off to his lab where he and his team of investigators spend hours, even days, studying the coronary arteries, the muscle, the valves. We were all particularly interested in this heart because it had functioned well as a transplant for over a decade before developing atherosclerosis. As transplant recipients were living longer, we were discovering that this so-called graft atherosclerosis was going to be the next major barrier to overcome. Only about fifty retransplants had ever been attempted, and this was Vanderbilt's first look at the old heart from such an operation. We knew that Jim was at greater risk than a first-time transplant patient. He would have a higher rate of rejection. Maybe Dr. Atkinson and his team of investigators could throw some light on why that was the case.

As I spoke to Jim Atkinson, I thought how important it was to be doing transplants at a major medical center such as Vanderbilt. Not only could we offer heart transplantation to those in need, but we could also conduct ongoing, aggressive research on the hearts we took out. This research would improve the field even further, so that someday we might be able to eliminate much of the heart disease we see today. In too many hospitals, that old heart we took out of Jim would be thrown in a wastebasket, never to be seen again. At Vanderbilt it was about to begin a journey that we hoped would unlock doors for others.

"Careful with this thing," I said. "It's got a treasured history."
He held open a plastic bag, and I picked up the severed organ and

slipped it inside. He twisted the bag closed and tied it tight.

"Dr. Atkinson," the circulating nurse said, "do you want me to label the bag?"

He laughed. "Don't think so. I'm not likely to get too many like this in the lab today."

"Or any day," Walter added.

Walter was suctioning excess blood from the chest cavity and placing the first stitch when Atkinson backed out the swinging doors carrying the old heart. I lifted the new one, cold and firm from its long ride in the ice-cold container, and lowered it deep into Jim Hayes's open chest.

"Is it right side up?" I asked.

Tom Wareing chuckled.

"I'm only half joking," I said. Because you had to rotate the heart to place the first suture line on its backside, even experienced heart surgeons had to pause to make sure they had the heart right side up. "Once at Stanford, one of the top guns was half-finished with the first suture line when he realized he had the heart in backwards. If it can happen there, it can happen to anybody." I told this story every time we did a transplant, the broader lesson being one that could not be overemphasized.

"Details," Walter said.

"That's right. Attention to detail."

The operation itself was straightforward, consisting of four anastomoses (a word derived from the Greek meaning "to join, mouth-to-mouth"), or points where we attached the new heart to the corresponding connections in Jim's body. I insisted on a strict order, always doing the operation in the exact same way, keeping it simple and orderly so that it became second nature, a technique with no room for mistakes.

First we connected the donor heart's left atrial chamber to what remained of Jim's left atrium, creating an entirely new chamber. Next, we sewed the two right atrial chambers together. Then we took the donor's aorta and attached it to Jim's, end to end. Finally, we anastomosed the pulmonary arteries. Walter sewed as

I positioned the heart and kept tension on the suture material to assure good apposition of the tissues.

"How was Florida?" Walter asked, as he quickly moved through the first suture line.

"Great. Full moon on the way down. Clear blue skies coming back. Beautiful. It was raining hard, though, when we left the hospital. The visibility was so poor, the helicopter pilot kept us low. Right about the height of your average downtown Tampa rooftop. You'd have just loved it." I poured a bucket of ice-cold saline on the heart as he continued sewing in order to keep it as cold as possible during its exposure to the hot operating-room lights.

"Right," he said. "The excitement. The thrills. Glad I missed it." He was shaking his head. Walter hated flying. He especially hated helicopters. Sometimes it literally made him sick. He didn't even like to talk about flying, so I of course always brought it up.

Stitching the heart took a little under an hour. The circulating nurse left the room occasionally to pick up more blood products or to drop off a blood-gas sample for the lab to analyze. Periodically a voice came over the OR intercom, "I've got blood gases for Hayes," and a nurse or the perfusionist or the anesthesiologist cocked an ear, even walked over to the intercom to take the information in case Walter or I missed it. When a nurse returned, her arms full of clear plastic packets of plasma, the anesthesiologist got up from his stool, clipboard in hand, and checked off the receipt of each packet on a form.

If we needed blood, the anesthesiologist would hook up a packet to one of the tubes running into Jim's body and suspend it high in the air on a pole at the head of the operating table. Behind him lay a fishing tackle box filled with bandages, alcohol swabs, needles, and various common drugs—epinephrine, heparin, furosemide, calcium chloride—anything the anesthesiologist might need at a moment's notice in the course of the operation.

Across the table, just behind Walter, was the little black accordion-like bellows of the ventilator, which had pumped up and down with each breath given to Jim before he was put on cardiopulmonary bypass. Now it remained collapsed, perfectly

42

motionless, as the heart-lung machine did the breathing for him.

Hunched over the surgical field, peering down into Jim's chest, watching Walter work in the bright patches lit by the head-lamps we both wore, I missed the medical student's arrival. But he was standing next to the anesthesiologist when I glanced up, his eyes wide above his mask. I didn't recognize him, but assumed he was rotating through on surgery and that he'd heard we were doing a transplant and gotten permission to observe.

"I'm Dr. Frist," I said. "That's Dr. Merrill over there. Have you ever seen a heart operation before?"

He shook his head and said, "No, sir."

"To this day I remember the first transplant I saw, standing right where you are," I said, flashing on the strangeness of it all, the confused jumble of tubes sticking out of the poor patient's chest, the operative field crowded with people huddled up against one another, the twirling wheels on the machines, the dark blood pouring down one tube into the heart-lung machine, the bright red blood flowing out another. "I felt lost."

The student caught my eyes before he quickly looked back to watch Walter as he was tying the first suture. I wondered if he was surprised by the size of the suture bites, the way I had been the first time I saw a transplant. The Stanford transplant fellow at the time, Doug Zusman, had telephoned me about three weeks after I had arrived in California and told me he was about to start a transplant. He said I should come over to watch because before long I would be in his shoes doing the operation.

Eager to learn the procedure, caught up in the drama of it all, I fought hard against the disappointment I felt with the technical aspects of the procedure itself. The huge suture bites, incorporating the full thickness of the heart's wall and its surrounding fat, seemed so rough and gross and inexact in contrast to the delicate, closely spaced sutures placed with the help of magnifying glasses in the more common coronary-artery bypass. Even the suture material seemed too big, almost like rope, in contrast to the thin, fine material we used in coronary-artery surgery.

"The sutures seem gigantic, don't they?" I asked the student. Another bucket of cold saline to the heart. He looked at me. "We take large bites," I said, "to prevent bleeding. To make sure the suture lines are tight enough to withstand the changing pressures of a beating heart. Remember, this heart has got to beat over 100,000 times a day for the next fifty years." He looked at me, seeming confused about what I was trying to say. "They guarantee a secure anastomosis and allow us to achieve hemostasis," I said, hopefully. He nodded that he understood.

Finished with the left atrium, Walter made his incision in the right. I stepped back a little and motioned surgical resident Tom Wareing in closer; as a resident in training it was important that he learn every step of the operation. "You ought to take a good look at this," I said. "We need to be especially careful to make the incision away from the sinus node." It was Dr. Christiaan Barnard who first emphasized the importance of keeping the incision away from that region of the heart that produced all its electrical activity. "That's Christiaan Barnard's only significant contribution to the field of heart transplantation," I said, repeating a phrase that floated around the Stanford operating rooms.

Tom's eyes wrinkled in a knowing smile. Those of us who came out of the Stanford program had little good to say about the man from South Africa who performed the world's first successful heart transplant. Norman Shumway had developed the procedure and spent years in the laboratory investigating the many facets of transplantation. With more than a little justification, we tended to give him the credit a fickle history had stolen for Barnard.

Walter had finished the anastomosis of the right atrium, leaving only the final connections of the two aortas and pulmonary arteries, when Jan Muirhead popped in to check on our progress.

"How's it going?" she said, standing on tiptoes next to Walter and peering over his shoulder into the chest.

"Moving right along," I said, cheerily. "We'll come off bypass in about an hour. Why don't you let Shirley know that everything's going along just fine."

I could picture Shirley sitting out there in the waiting room, curled up on the end of one of the nondescript brown couches, her dark, penetrating eyes staring off at the wall, ignoring the inanities of whatever soap opera happened to be playing on the television slung from the ceiling. There would be others in there, too, waiting for news from different operations, all of them wearing that same stare. From time to time, they might talk to each other, exchange quick life stories, try to give each other a little sympathy or a little encouragement. But they would never really break free of the stare, their attention would never be far from the corner where any second now a doctor or nurse might appear, dressed in scrubs, surgical mask dropped down below the chin, bringing a report of an operation.

As troublesome as the stare was, the glance up at you when you walked into the room was worse. Every head snapped up, each expression a mixture of fear and questioning, the eyes searching your face for some clue that would tell them whether you had come for them, and—if you had—what kind of news you brought.

During a transplant operation, Jan stayed in constant touch with the family of the patient, giving them brief reports on the progress of the operation, trying for just a moment, often with just a word or two, to break through the fearful isolation in which they waited. She did it well, and her rapport with the families testified to that. Tonight, of all nights, Shirley needed to see Jan, to feel some connection through her with Jim's strange, unseen, frightening ordeal. And tonight, so far, the news was all good.

Walter and I trimmed the aorta of the donor heart, sculpturing the closest fit possible with Jim's aorta. The medical student's eagerness was palpable as he peered over the head of the table to get a better look. Through the end of the opened aorta, we could see the valve.

"Look at the leaflets," I said to the student. "So delicate."

Was that irony I saw in Walter's glance? We sewed the two aortas together, and I turned to the perfusionist, saying "Let's warm 'em up."

During the operation, we had cooled the blood in the heart-lung machine by about twenty degrees to slow the patient's metabolism; this would decrease the body's demand for oxygen and would preserve the vitality of the heart-muscle cells. Once we'd hooked up the aortas, we reheated the oxygenated blood as it flowed through the machine and into the coronary arteries that fed the heart.

Slowly, gently, the heart warmed up. Walter placed the final sutures in the pulmonary artery. The rich, warm blood began pouring into the new heart, feeding its millions of cells that had been starving for three hours and twenty minutes. For hearts, we could allow four hours of ischemic time. After that, there was the risk that too many of the heart-muscle cells had been irreversibly damaged for the heart to work properly. But tonight we were well within the limit, and my own heart began to beat faster as we finished the final suturing. We were all waiting for the first quick beat, the moment of truth when the new heart would begin to pump blood through Jim's body.

I knew in every fiber of my body that it was coming, and I feared in every recess of my mind that it wouldn't.

And then Walter said, "Look!" The room was quiet, all eyes on the field.

The limp heart began to quiver. We just stood and watched. I held my breath. I thought about reaching for the defibrillator paddles behind me, connected to the machine that you see doctors on television using to blast cardiac-arrest patients back to life. Often we used these, at a much lower voltage, to start up a transplanted heart or to shock it into a regular rhythm if it began to fibrillate.

But not this time. For suddenly, amidst all the quivering and all the focused attention, the heart jumped, then began thumping slowly and rhythmically. The squeezing contractions were strong and regular. Once more, the miracle had occurred. I felt good and pure, sure that God was in heaven and all was well down below.

Jim Hayes was alive again.

Part Two

CHIMERAS

1

It was morning before we had Jim patched up and off to the intensive-care unit, where he would spend the next three or four days in isolation. He would be carefully monitored, meticulously protected from contact with bacteria and viruses—organisms innocuous to us but potentially deadly to him. He would be tested repeatedly and subjected to a rigid protocol of multiple drugs to suppress his immune system. At this moment, that system was his worst enemy, more dangerous even than his body's reaction to the brutal insult of surgery.

After the operation was over, I left Jim in the cardiac recovery room and went to the waiting room to see Shirley. All night and morning long, Jan had reassured her that Jim was fine and that the operation was proceeding as we had hoped. But for those who waited, only the surgeon's word could really bring them peace. They had literally put their loved one's life in his hands, and only he—like a priest in matters spiritual—had the authority to utter truth. They needed my benediction. Whenever possible, I offered it.

Spotting me through the door, Shirley hurriedly struggled up out of the sofa. She shot me the Glance, and I smiled. I knew she was interested in one and only one thing: Is Jim alive? Is Jim all right? The details of the process, the trip to Florida, the removal of the heart, the moment it began to beat, the separation from the bypass machine, all the events and worries that had pressed on me over the last twenty-four hours would mean nothing to her.

What she needed was the telling headline, the short, sensational news story, but I had to be careful. Transplant surgery is so different from all other surgery. Most surgeons fix something broken, take out an angry appendix, lop off an offensive growth,

49

remove a nagging gallbladder. By doing so, they eliminate the underlying problem. They expected uneventful recoveries, fast, worry-free returns to normal life. Heart transplants involved not a single problem, but a series of smaller constantly changing problems that never allowed the surgeon to relax or even think about dropping his defenses. With every piece of good news, there came a warning.

"Things are coming along fine," I said. "Just as I expected. Under the circumstances, Jim is doing extremely well, and I'm pleased. Everything has fallen into place. But as we discussed, these first twenty-four hours are critical, and there is a chance, perhaps one in ten, that we'll have to go back to the operating room today or tomorrow if the bleeding doesn't slow down. Many things can still slip up on us. We will keep a very close watch on him tonight and tomorrow as he wakes up. If anything happens that worries me, I will let you know immediately. But right now, everything looks perfect."

She hung on every word, nodding now and again, watching. As I talked I could see her features relax, could see the understanding dawning that the ordeal was fast drawing to a close. Near tears, she almost smiled.

"When can I see him?" she asked.

"As soon as the nurses get him settled in," I said. "Within an hour, but don't count on too much. He'll be breathing through a tube in his mouth, not much of a conversationalist. And his face will be swollen. There'll be lines and tubes everywhere. But that's all normal."

We talked for a bit longer, and when I turned to go, she put her hand on my arm, and said, "Thank you, Dr. Frist. Bless you."

I appreciated Shirley's heartfelt gratitude; it was one of the things that made being a surgeon worthwhile. But as I walked away, I thought to myself how misplaced in some ways that gratitude was. Shumway had always stressed that the surgeon's operative skill was truly the minor part of a successful transplant. Jim Hayes would survive because someone had stumbled onto cyclosporine a few years back, because a nurse and organ-procurement coordinator in Florida had had the temerity to intrude on a family's grief, and because Jim Hayes had the ability to walk the medical tightrope we would string for him across the rest of his life.

The satisfaction I felt was more like that of a good quarterback than a great surgeon. It was the teamwork, the calling of the plays, the attention to details, the timing and execution of a master plan that made for a successful operation. The four suture lines we had placed to hold the heart together were just that—four suture lines. And later, as I was changing out of my scrubs in the surgeon's locker room, more than a bit weary, I found myself running back over the night, analyzing it just the way a quarterback would review each play of the big game he had just played.

Had I been too hard on the anesthesiologist in Florida? After all, the heart was fine, despite his complacency. No, I decided, the heart was simply too precious to risk losing it needlessly. We had over two thousand people each year who were dying of heart trouble and waiting to be called for a transplant. Last year, we had only found fifteen hundred hearts for them. Simple arithmetic meant that too many of them, nearly a third, would die waiting.

Organ donation had slacked off, partly because of the lowered speed limit and seat-belt laws, which had dramatically reduced the number of people who died in accidents. I was glad for that, of course. But it was a fact that some 25,000 people whose organs could be used for transplantation still died in the slaughter on our highways. There could be plenty of organs for everyone waiting for hearts, for lungs, for kidneys, for livers, for corneas, if only the accident victims' relatives would donate those organs—and if only my fellow doctors would ask for them.

Part of the problem was that the average person did not understand brain death. I could see why. For thousands of years, you were dead when your heart stopped beating and your lungs quit breathing. Your body stiffened up, your lips drew back in a ghastly grin, your eyes stared glazed and blank, your skin paled—you *were* dead and you *looked* dead.

These days you died when your brain stopped functioning,

when all activity in the brain that gave the word *life* any rational meaning quit beyond hope of revival. When the brain was destroyed, you were dead. You were not asleep. You were not in a coma. You would never get up and walk around. But now we could run a plastic tube down your windpipe and hook you up to a ventilator. For quite some time, while you were dead, your heart would continue to beat, your lungs would pump oxygen into your blood. Your kidneys, liver, pancreas would all work, though not without the machines. The trouble was, you didn't look dead.

It was a matter of perception, not reality.

Relatives came in, saw the body of their son or daughter or husband or wife hooked up to the ventilator appearing more alive than Jim Hayes did right now. Naturally, they wanted to believe that everything was all right. Sure, the body might have a bruise here and there, but otherwise the accident didn't seem to have done much damage. As soon as the doctors finished, the patient would climb out of bed, say "Good morning," and everybody would pile in the car, head home, and take up life again.

And even if the physician explained clearly just how dead the loved one was, it took a while for the family to accept it, to feel the loss, to begin grieving for someone who was so alive at dinner the night before. Someone who even now looked as if he were enjoying a long, peaceful rest.

The doctors could pull the plug to prove that the body was in fact dead. The rise and fall of the chest would stop. The heart would become flaccid. The traditional signs of death would quickly appear. But it was rarely necessary. Eventually almost everyone did understand brain death, abstract as it was. And most people, once they came to understand it, were willing to donate the organs of their loved ones *if they were asked*. I had back on my desk a document that I thought about almost constantly. It was a Gallup poll on organ donation. It showed that more than eighty percent of those polled said that they would consider donating the organs of a brain-dead spouse or sibling if we asked them to do so.

But we weren't asking. At least, not often enough.

The problem in large part came down to doctors. There were enough potential donors to save every single patient who would die without a heart transplant. No organized Western religion opposed donation. If properly approached, families usually did not object. Yet people—my patients, my friends—died daily because doctors, entrusted by society to care for its ills and its health, too often felt awkward and uncomfortable approaching grieving families.

Many doctors, especially in rural areas, didn't know much about the relatively new field of transplantation. They thought that this miracle cure was some kind of chimera. Most were trained long before heart transplants were possible; some were unaware of our successes and ignorant of the important role they played in this process by finding potential donors. Others, after striving valiantly to save a patient, simply walked away in despair when the patient died. Physicians were trained to save lives, to thwart death, not to petition a family for the loved one's heart. To doctors, death—even brain death—meant defeat. They saw the body as a corpse, not a potential donor. Losing a patient damaged their self-esteem. They couldn't make themselves ask.

Many doctors would rather avoid talking about brain death. At best, they left it to a nurse, an intern, or an organ-procurement coordinator. At worst, they forced the family to bear the entire decision of whether or not to take the patient off the machines.

One survey haunted me more than all the rest. A marketing firm had polled doctors about their reluctance to approach potential donor families. A number of those surveyed admitted that they felt they couldn't spare the time to explain the situation to a family because it did not bring them any additional fees. They suggested that they would be more willing to do so if they could get a percentage of the money brought in from the organ transplant.

But I truly did not believe that the refusal grew merely from excessive self-esteem or unseemly greed. It was more subtle than that. Transplants had literally revolutionized medicine. For most of man's existence, when a heart or liver or other organ quit functioning, the entire body died. Now, that was no longer true. That simple fact, tied to the shortage of available organs, turned the medical profession on its head. Gone almost overnight was the bedrock verity of traditional medicine, which said that the physician was first, foremost, and always the complete advocate for his patient. The decision I had made last night to give Jim Hayes a new heart and to keep another man waiting was a decision that no doctor ever had to make twenty years ago.

And it had not been my decision alone. Even before the phone call pulled me away from Harrison's bedtime story, data about the available donor heart had been run through a new national computer network set up by federal law. The computer had determined that I could retrieve the heart for one of my patients based on a set of criteria established by law, not just medical criteria, but time and geographic criteria as well.

The whole process went against the grain of what most doctors understood as sound medical practice. It was almost impossible for an older doctor, for a more traditional doctor, perhaps for any doctor outside transplantation to embrace the notion that his own patient, whom he had referred for a transplant, might have to die because some other doctor, some faceless, nameless physician a thousand miles away, had a patient who better fit the imposed and sometimes arbitrary standards plugged into an impersonal computer.

Most doctors fiercely resented the federal law that now required hospitals, if they wished to keep their Medicare reimbursements, to ask the families of brain-dead patients to donate organs. For decades doctors had worked independently. They were not used to being told what to do, and the required-notification law seemed a step on the road toward socialized medicine. Without the support of the doctors, the law itself had little impact. Being a doctor, I understood how they felt, just as I empathized with families who were confused by the idea of brain death.

The governments of Sweden, France, and Greece, among others, operated under what was called presumed consent. Unless a family expressly objected or there was concrete evidence to the contrary, doctors presumed that a brain-dead accident victim had consented to the use of his organs for transplants. How radically different was the United States. Even if a potential donor had previously signed a donor card, no U.S. hospital or doctor or procurement agency would touch the body without first obtaining verbal consent from the next of kin. The only way we could retrieve organs in this country was by asking relatives for permission. Maybe, I thought, we should learn from other countries and adopt presumed-consent laws. Relying on our so-called traditional American voluntarism was failing miserably as people around the country died daily waiting for organs.

Since doctors did not ask, and nurses were often reluctant to do so, more and more hospitals had come to rely on the coordinators from the organ-procurement agencies. People like Rusty and Nancy made the system work. They encouraged—occasionally gently badgered—neurosurgeons for identification of potential donors and declarations of brain death. They faced grieving, sometimes hostile, families, knowing that time was against them, that every moment consent was delayed made the organs less and less stable.

With considerable tact and talent, these coordinators explained brain death and the social value and private satisfaction of donation to relatives who usually did not know the wishes of their loved ones concerning organ donation, who were reluctant to act without knowing, whose natural inclination was to say no and avoid the entire issue. They fought fears spawned by movies like *Coma* and assured relatives that absolutely everything that could be done for the potential donor had been done. They assuaged family worries about the funeral, reassuring relatives that the process would cause no delays and the loved one's body would look as if it had come from a mortuary. They reviewed how the whole procedure worked, made it clear that the donor family could not choose who got the organs, and discouraged the family from trying to discover or to contact the recipients to prevent emotionally charged and potentially damaging relationships from developing. They helped the family through its bereavement, doing all they could to shield the family from a sometimes excessively inquisitive press.

They arranged to have the donor properly cared for, sitting by the body as it was taken off the ventilator to demonstrate that the donor would not miraculously revive on his own. They obtained the necessary data to determine if the various organs were satisfactory for transplantation, helped manage the donor's blood pressure and fluid requirements, obtained the appropriate consents, and initiated the computerized search for the most suitable recipients for the heart, kidneys, and liver.

They contacted the transplant surgeons. They coordinated transportation for the organ runs. They transported the organs. Not infrequently, they burned themselves out. They got too close to the donor families, saw the tragic ends of too many young lives, ate too much fast food, slept in too many strange places, spent too little time at home. Hooked on the drama, telephone junkies, medical romantics, they found themselves of necessity growing callous or indifferent or simply steely nerved and professional, suffering all the drawbacks of being a surgeon yet garnering few of the rewards.

They became neither especially powerful nor respected. Needy donor families fed upon them. Many surgeons found them irritating, especially in the operating room, where they occasionally rushed matters and got in the way. If they knew what was good for them, they steered clear of potential recipients to protect themselves emotionally. Thus organ recipients often had only a vague notion of the pivotal role the coordinators played and saved their profuse gratitude for the surgeon and the transplant program's nurses. Hospital personnel treated the coordinators as outsiders, intruders. Few people knew what they did or much cared.

But the pay was OK, and they saved a few lives.

As I closed my locker and straightened my tie, I thought about trying to find Rusty and Nancy. If I'd been a drinking man, I could have invited them to a local bistro, ordered a round, and toasted them and their ilk, the unsung heros of the transplant world. Instead, I thought I'd ask them to split a pizza with me. But by the time I headed out, they were nowhere to be seen.

2

Over the next few days, I kept close watch on Jim Hayes's condition. I generally made rounds by six in the morning, while the hospital was still quiet. That way I could concentrate on my patients. Each morning I would drop by Jim's isolation room, review his chart, quickly examine him from head to toe, and give him a few vital words of encouragement.

I relied on the nurses for most of my information, a habit I picked up first from my father and then from Norman Shumway. I saw Jim briefly each morning, but the nurses lived with him, minute by minute, every day and every night. Their observations of changes as subtle as mood shifts or as clear as variations in heart rate were the key to Jim's post-op care. The nurses made sure that the hundreds of tests I routinely ordered—to check Jim's blood chemistry, to track his kidney function, to search for impending infections—were carried out. They diligently monitored the results, bringing to my attention anything out of line.

I knew that Jim would almost certainly go through a period of rejection during the first several weeks after his operation. Nearly all transplant recipients do. After all, rejection was nothing more than the human body trying to cure itself of an invasion by alien tissue. Jim's body greeted his new heart like an unwelcome and hostile foreigner. For him to go on living, we had to subdue his body's attack against this invader, and we did that by judiciously crippling his immune system.

The powerful immunosuppressive drugs we fed into Jim each day not only prevented his body from rejecting the new heart but, much to our disadvantage, also stripped him of important natural protection against simple infections like the common cold. Such was the transplant surgeon's Catch-22.

*   *   *

Shumway had struggled mightily with this dilemma in the dark ages of transplantation before the discovery of cyclosporine. At the time, practically everyone else had given up on transplanting hearts. But not Shumway. The "old man," as his residents affectionately called him, had a vision—and he made it real.

He came out of the University of Michigan as an undergraduate during World War II and joined the army with plans to become an engineer. But the government needed doctors and transferred a number of engineering students, Shumway among them, into pre-med. He got his M.D. from Vanderbilt in 1949, finished his stint with the armed services, and took a fellowship at Minnesota, known as the mecca for training cardiac surgeons in those days. In 1958, he wound up at the Stanford Medical Center as a heart surgeon.

When Shumway arrived, the medical school was still in San Francisco. Amidst some controversy, it soon moved to more rural Palo Alto, about an hour to the south. There Shumway and his assistant, Dr. Richard Lower, spent their time in a tiny, primitive laboratory experimenting with dogs to make open-heart surgery safer. One afternoon they had removed the heart from a dog, keeping the animal alive on a heart-lung bypass machine and cooling the heart in saline solution, when Shumway decided to put the heart back in, reconnect it, and see what happened. (He had taken the heart out in the first place so he could work on it without straining his back by leaning over to work inside the animal's chest cavity.) His experiment worked. The heart began to beat on its own.

For nearly a decade, Shumway and Lower conducted exhaustive laboratory research to perfect the surgical procedure. They dissected and defined the physiology of the transplanted heart and determined the most accurate and sensitive ways to diagnose and treat rejection and infection.

The concept of transplanting organs and tissues was not new. Skin grafting, the simplest kind of tissue transplant, had been practiced with success for centuries, but it only worked with skin from the patient's own body. Skin taken from someone else shriveled up and flaked off within a matter of days.

During World War II, a brilliant young biologist in England named Peter Medawar became fascinated with immunology when he was assigned the task of saving badly burned airmen. Frustrated by his lack of success, he went back to the laboratory after the war. There, he performed the animal experiments that defined the fundamental immunologic and genetic phenomena on which much of transplantation is based.

Medawar established the existence of the second-set response. The first time someone received a skin graft, he would reject the transplanted skin in seven days. If a second graft was attempted on the same person, he would reject it in three days. The body had built up a specific response to the foreign tissue that cut the rejection time in half. Later, he discovered an immunologic weakness in the immune response of very young babies. For a brief period in their early lives, babies' underdeveloped immune systems allowed them to accept transplants without rejecting them. Medawar's research excited the scientific world. He eventually won the Nobel Prize in medicine and physiology, and received a knighthood. Based on his findings, clinical transplantation was born.

In a landmark operation on December 23, 1954, Boston surgeon Joseph Murray demonstrated that an organ transplant was indeed possible. He boldly removed one of the two healthy kidneys from Ronald Herrick and placed it in Richard, his identical twin brother, who was dying because both of his kidneys were failing. Because they were identical twins, their tissues matched perfectly, and Ronald's immune system did not recognize his brother's transplanted kidney as foreign. There was no rejection. People could live with only one kidney, so whole organ transplantation became a reality for the first time. And Boston became the world center for transplanting kidneys between identical twins.

Before long, kidney surgeons began to have some success with transplants between closely matched but unrelated donors by using radical techniques, such as total body irradiation, to cripple the immune system. Later, they developed a cocktail of drugs—mostly steroids—that suppressed the recipient's immune system, pacifying its natural, typically violent reaction to transplanted foreign organs. In 1959, researchers performing animal experiments discovered that the agent azathioprine modified the immune response more selectively. In 1963, they used this agent in a human kidney transplant; the recipient survived for a year.

Even with these successes in immunosuppression, there were problems. The steroids created huge mood swings, even brief periods of psychosis; they puffed up a patient's cheeks like a balloon; sometimes they destroyed bone tissue. The irradiation so effectively inhibited the immune system that many patients died of overwhelming infections. The first two patients receiving azathioprine died from its toxic effects.

But over time, scientists like Shumway and his team modified and improved the various immunosuppressant regimens developed for kidney transplant patients. Soon Shumway felt confident, based on his extensive and careful preparatory research, that he could control rejection sufficiently to transplant a human heart. An artificial kidney could keep someone with failing kidneys alive even without a transplant, but there was no such device for people with failing hearts. They died, sometimes suddenly, sometimes slowly and painfully. Despite the side effects of the immunosuppressants, these drugs offered an alternative. In the November 1967 issue of the *Journal of the American Medical Association*, Shumway formally announced his plans for transplanting a human heart.

Meanwhile, Dr. Lower had gone from Stanford to the Medical College of Virginia, where a visiting doctor from South Africa named Christiaan Barnard was observing kidney transplants. Barnard had known Shumway at Minnesota, and he sat in on one of Lower's canine heart transplants. The procedure fascinated him, and he returned to South Africa dreaming of historic possibilities.

The operation Shumway had described in *JAMA* was delayed when the first available donor heart was unsuitable for his patient. Back home in South Africa, Barnard seized the opportunity. Shumway, still waiting for an appropriate donor, picked up his morning paper on December 3, 1967, and read the news from Cape Town.

There was Louis Washkansky, a fifty-five-year-old grocer, smiling beside the young, handsome Barnard and sporting a new heart taken from a twenty-three-year-old woman killed in an automobile accident. "I'm the new Frankenstein," Washkansky said. He died eighteen days later of pneumonia.

But it was too late for Shumway. The operation had fired the public's imagination like no other breakthrough in the history of medicine. Barnard became a world celebrity overnight. He was invited to lunch by the president of the United States, and the press asked his opinion not only on every imaginable medical matter, but also on totally unrelated political and social issues as well.

Surgeons throughout the United States felt robbed. Almost all of the basic research behind the procedure had been carried out in this country, most of it under Shumway's auspices. Yet the credit was going to a little-known man in South Africa who knew almost nothing about the vital underlying animal research. Shumway put it in perspective for me many years later when he said, "I remember my conversation with Chris just after that first transplant. His only interest was to learn from us as quickly as possible how to diagnose rejection of the transplanted heart."

Soon others, even some who had been the most skeptical, rushed to perform heart transplants. Pioneering heart and vascular surgeon Dr. Michael DeBakey, known as the Texas Tornado, had long been a proponent of artificial hearts as the more likely approach to replacing failing hearts. But when Dr. Denton Cooley, DeBakey's former assistant and then his biggest rival, became transplantation's most vocal supporter, DeBakey too tried his hand at the operation.

Within a year, the irrepressible and technically acclaimed Cooley had—in typical Texas and Cooley fashion—transplanted more hearts than any other physician in the world, proclaiming his feelings of "exhilaration" with a procedure that could "renovate an old carcass." Cooley kept a high profile, and when he released pictures of patients lying in bed, dying of heart disease, juxtaposed with shots of them back at work after transplantation, many thousands of people with heart disease took hope—prematurely, as it turned out.

Through all the feverish activity and giddy promises, Norman Shumway kept his head. Those at Stanford who worked with Shumway were amazed at his attitude toward the cruel twist of fate that robbed him of the public recognition he so deserved for the years spent in the laboratory establishing a sound, scientific basis for human heart transplantation. An unassuming and personable man who actively avoided the spotlight and always gave credit to those around him, Shumway showed absolutely no sign of bitterness.

Shumway performed the first successful heart transplant in the United States a month after Barnard's operation, though this patient too lived only a short while—fifteen days. When the subject came up, Shumway would always say with a smile "What was the name of the second man to fly solo across the Atlantic?" In fact, he claimed that it had all worked out for the best, that the notoriety would have been troublesome, that it would have interfered with his carefully controlled approach to basic research.

The initial clamor to perform the dramatic and radical new procedure seemed to grow into a world-wide epidemic. But the postoperative antirejection procedures applied to kidneys proved less successful with hearts. For the most part, heart surgeons had no experience with transplantation, much less with immunosuppressive chemotherapy. Before too many months, most of the patients who received the first heart transplants took a turn for the worse. Fluid flooded their chests, they began to suffocate, their livers bloated, their bodies rejected their new hearts, and they died, one by one. By 1970, only 23 of the 166 people who had received heart transplants were still alive.

Headlines began to appear in newspapers across the country:
"Heart Surgery Is Direct Killing—the Vatican."
"Must They Play God to Work Miracles?"
"New Heart Operations Are 'a Crime' says Nobel Surgeon."
"Too Soon for Heart Swaps Says Surgeon."
Everyone's results were disastrous—everyone's but Shum-

way's. Nine of the twenty-six patients he had transplanted were still alive; though his mortality rate was far from ideal, it was clearly superior to the disastrous eighty-five percent rate overall. Denton Cooley, the conspicuous leader of the worldwide transplant frenzy, had for years claimed the surgeon's motto should be "cut well, tie well, get well." His credo, however, had not worked with transplants. Within a year, he had lost almost all of his transplanted patients.

And for the first time Shumway, who normally avoided interviews, spoke out publicly. He called Cooley's prescription for success naive and said if transplantation had been primarily a matter of cutting and sewing, all the people who had received transplants would have survived. The real problems, Shumway knew all along, came with the care of the recipient after surgery.

The demonstrated mortality rate was simply too high. Most surgeons who had jumped on the transplant bandwagon abandoned the procedure. Cooley, in a news conference, announced that he would no longer perform the procedure. He explained what was by then obvious, "I have done all that I can do as a surgeon. It remains for the immunologists and biologists to unravel the mysteries that have limited our work." Teaching hospitals and research centers declared heart transplants too experimental. But Shumway refused to give up. He never altered his pace. He simply continued his systematic exploration.

Shumway and Lower perfected the now standard transplant technique which is really a partial transplant of the heart. This was basically the same operation we had performed on Jim Hayes.

The heart is pear shaped and hollow, weighing about ten ounces. It is a bundle of muscle strips wound in all directions, the way yarn can be wound around a hollow ball. Muscles can only contract, pulling themselves shorter; that's all the heart does— contract with a jerk.

Inside, the heart is really two pumps. Imagine a four-room duplex with two rooms on each side. The upstairs rooms are called the atria, the downstairs rooms the ventricles. The two rooms on the right are separated from the two rooms on the left by a wall. The two halves of the duplex are absolutely private. No door exists between them. But each upstairs and downstairs is a single unit, and a trap door opens out of each atrium into the ventricle below. The door opens only one way—down. Whatever goes through can't come back up.

Blood collects in the upper rooms. When the atria are full, the heart muscle contracts, the two trap doors swing open, the blood pours down into the lower rooms. At the same time, the blood already in the two ventricles is pumped out of the duplex altogether. The blood that collected in the right atrium was blood carrying wastes from the body. The right ventricle pumps that blood into the lungs to dispose of its wastes and pick up a new supply of oxygen. The blood that collected in the left atrium came from the lungs. The left ventricle pumps it through arteries to the rest of the body, where it delivers the load of oxygen.

Shumway cut the upper rooms, the atria or collecting chambers, in half and took out the two lower rooms, the ventricles or pumping chambers, leaving the upper back wall of the duplex intact. He then tailored the new heart to match what remained of the upper rooms. The importance of the technique was that it simplified the number of connections between blood vessels, thereby shortening the operation.

Shumway had found a brilliant assistant named Dr. Ed Stinson, known in the Stanford medical community as the mastermind behind heart transplants. Stinson helped Shumway develop and define the donor and recipient criteria that increased patients' odds for survival. Together they tirelessly experimented with immunosuppression, ultimately developing a three-drug combination therapy that included steroids, azathioprine, and RATG. This last was rabbit antithymocyte globulin, a drug that another Stanford physician produced locally, allegedly in his garage several miles off campus. This drug helped Shumway and Stinson immensely in their constant seesaw battle to balance prevention of rejection against the risk of infection and to reverse the inevitable episodes of rejection when they occurred.

Finally in the early 1970s, Shumway and Stinson supervised Dr. Philip Caves's development of a technique to monitor rejection that would prove invaluable in solving postsurgical problems. Using a small catheter called a bioptome threaded through a vein in the patient's neck, Shumway's team could routinely obtain small pieces of heart tissue for direct examination under the microscope. With this method, they could detect rejection long before the patient got sick and clinical signs appeared—a revolutionary breakthrough.

Shumway—still chasing his dream one step at a time—continued to transplant hearts. He worked without encouragement from his peers, often in the face of their criticism. For the most part, they thought he had set for himself an impossible task.

He pioneered new ethical and legal grounds as well. Stanford hospital administrators had entered into an agreement with the local Santa Clara county coroner not to use homicide victims as donors. But in 1973, when the neighboring Alameda County district attorney called Shumway to offer a heart on behalf of a homicide victim's next of kin, Shumway accepted it. At that point no one had ever gone outside of the recipient's hospital to remove a heart and transport it back. But since the local agreement prevented him from moving the body to Stanford, Shumway sent his team to Oakland to get the organ. It was the first time that anyone had tried "distant" heart procurement.

The man accused of killing the donor dragged Shumway and company to court. His attorney claimed that the surgeons, not the defendant, had ultimately caused the victim's death. For the first time a jury had to decide the legality of brain death. They established it as a true definition of death, which set an important precedent in California.

Because of Shumway's persistence, Jim Hayes—facing certain death at twenty-three—had someplace to turn in 1976. And because Shumway stuck with it, the medical profession had a vast amount of accumulated laboratory and clinical experience with which to stage the dramatic comeback of heart transplantation when cyclosporine was introduced on an experimental basis in 1980.

In 1969 a microbiologist from Sandoz, a Swiss pharmaceutical firm, was on vacation in southern Norway. Since the discovery of penicillin, drug companies were always on the lookout for bacterial microbes that would make good antibiotics. They encouraged their employees, even on vacation, to dig among the moss and lichen of the world on the off chance that something might turn up. So the microbiologist dug up a soil sample from an isolated plateau and took it home to study in his laboratory in Basel. This time something did turn up: an organic compound no one had ever seen before. Sandoz dubbed it cyclosporine.

Laboratory tests soon proved that cyclosporine was not much of an antibiotic, and the company accordingly lost interest. The compound did, however, have some properties that intrigued another Sandoz scientist named Jean-François Borel, who had gotten his Ph.D. in immunogenetics from the University of Wisconsin. He ran a second series of tests and discovered that cyclosporine had tremendous power to suppress the immune system. Moreover, it did not kill just any immune cell, as steroids and azathioprine did, but instead wiped out the T lymphocytes, the killer cells that are sent out in response to foreign tissue.

If his results held up, Borel realized, he had discovered a unique drug that could fight rejection while leaving the rest of the immune system capable of preventing most infections. Organ transplantation would no longer be a chimerical hope but a palpable reality. But transplantation had fallen into such disrepute that Sandoz at first refused to fund the research necessary to prove the drug's therapeutic value.

Borel had very little cyclosporine on hand; it was all of the substance that existed in the world. He tried, without success, to interest European doctors in its peculiar properties. He then gave as much as he could spare to a few British clinicians. Small as the sample was, they managed to achieve encouraging results with it in animal experiments. Those results caused a stir in the medical profession, and Sandoz gave a tentative go-ahead on production. In 1980, after several false starts (one of cyclosporine's side effects was liver damage and certain dosages proved toxic in rats) both Dr. Tom Starzl, who had pioneered liver and kidney transplantation at the University of Colorado, and Norman Shumway received the drug for experimental use. Based on their own extensive laboratory and clinical experience, they combined cyclosporine with steroids and other drugs and began to achieve amazing results.

In 1983, the Food and Drug Administration approved the use of cyclosporine combined with steroids for all transplant patients. The revolution was underway. Between 1980 and 1989, the number of heart transplants increased some twenty times. Transplant centers sprang up everywhere. Organ-procurement organizations emerged. The field blossomed.

I was at Stanford with Shumway and Stinson during the early cyclosporine era. I remember the team's ecstatic response to the initial results we achieved as we switched most of the transplant patients, like Jim Hayes, onto cyclosporine. Even before I arrived, cyclosporine, with all its immunosuppressive advantages over earlier chemotherapy, had allowed the calm, methodical, even stubborn Shumway to push beyond mere heart transplants to the transplantation of heart and lungs together.

We were a long way from the morning Louis Washkansky had declared himself the new Frankenstein monster. A medical symbol for transplantation was, in fact, the chimera. For classical scholars, the chimera was a monster, a mythological, fire-breathing beast with a lion's head, a goat's body, and a serpent's tail. Genetically, a chimera was an organism composed of two or more distinct tissues or an artificially produced individual having tissues of several species. Commonly, chimera implied something ineffable, an idle fancy, an impossible dream.

As I stood outside Jim's isolation room, washing my hands with a special lotion to kill germs, carefully shielding my mouth and nose with a surgical mask, peering in through the window at Jim, huge tubes sticking out his chest and artificial lines connecting his veins to suspended plastic bags, I thought about all that had gone into bringing him to this point. He did seem something of an impossible dream, made up of medical history, personal tragedy, courage, a lot of hope, some skill, a good deal of chance, but real, alive—one of my tender chimeras.

3

My new chimera had arrived in the recovery room a cold, pale, motionless body, looking hardly alive, intravenous lines flowing out of his veins, a tube running from his mouth to the ventilator. Two huge chest tubes lay along his new heart, sticking out through the skin beneath his ribs. They suctioned blood that leaked from around the sutures holding his heart together; the blood flowed into a bubbling canister at the foot of his bed.

Every four hours, as the blood filled the suction machine, the nurses emptied it back into Jim's veins to cut down on the number of blood transfusions we had to give him. In this way we minimized Jim's risk of contracting hepatitis or AIDS. The latter was especially unlikely; the chance of getting AIDS from a blood transfusion in Tennessee in the late 1980s was something like 1 in 10,000.

Immediately after Jim arrived, two special-care nurses went to work on him, adjusting the various infusion pumps, turning him from side to side every thirty minutes, and pounding his back as physical therapy for his lungs and his swollen, sore, cut-up chest. They put him on the routine medicines we give all our postoperative heart-transplant recipients—Isuprel, dopamine, antibiotics, and the immunosuppressive drugs.

The Isuprel made Jim's heart beat faster than normal and allowed his blood to flow more easily through his lungs, insuring that his new heart functioned perfectly. The low dosage of dopamine improved the flow of blood to his kidneys, encouraging them to work properly and rid his body of excess fluid and metabolic waste. We continued both drugs for five days.

For the first twenty-four hours we deluged his body with huge doses of steroids to shut down his immune system and prevent the acute rejection that had so plagued heart transplants in the early years. At the same time, we pumped him full of two antibiotics for forty-eight hours to keep infections from invading his body along the lines and tubes that pierced his skin. For most patients this would have been the beginning of the balancing act worked out so delicately by Stinson and Shumway, but Jim had been on the seesaw most of his adult life.

As I told Shirley, we watched Jim especially carefully that first night. Because of his previous surgery, Jim had numerous adhesions around his heart, all of which we had cut apart during the operation and all of which could continue to bleed post-op.

Most of my patients bled a fair amount after surgery, albeit for different reasons than Jim. Many of them received Coumadin, a blood thinner that kept them from forming clots in their old hearts. Those diseased organs, big and baggy, took up a lot of room in their chests, and when we put in the healthy new hearts they would be too small to take up all the space. Blood often accumulated there. Often a patient's liver—which normally helped blood to coagulate—failed to function properly because the old heart had not been able to pump enough blood to nourish it. Thin blood made bleeding one of the risks of transplant surgery.

Much to my relief, Jim's bleeding slowed, and he passed the first night uneventfully. Six hours after he arrived in the isolation room, Jim began to wake up. The nurses were already weaning him off the ventilator. At first, the machine cycled eight breaths into him every minute, but every hour or so the nurses turned down the ventilator until Jim was breathing on his own. As he came out of his deep sleep, he would try to talk, but the breathing tube that passed through his vocal cords into his windpipe made that impossible. When he woke up, he chewed on the endotracheal tube like a big, heavy cigar, anxiously waiting for us to get rid of the annoying device. Awaking from the forced dream-like sleep of anesthesia was bad enough; adding the discomfort of a foot-long tube stuck in his throat only heightened his frustration.

Fully awake and breathing on his own, he clearly wanted to say something as soon as I pulled the endotracheal tube out.

"It's about time, Doc. What are you trying to do, kill me?" he blurted out with his first gasp, trying to laugh.

Not long after we extubated him, the nurses removed the nasogastric tube. This tube, which ran through his nose down the back of his throat and through his esophagus, had kept his stomach free of air and fluids so that Jim could not vomit and aspirate his stomach contents when we pumped anesthetic gases into him. That same afternoon, Jim got the last of the large steroid doses.

During those first three days, I also used a Nashville version of the rabbit antithymocyte globulin, the immunosuppressive drug that Shumway and company had made in the Stanford garage. Instead of injecting it into Jim's thigh muscles, as we had in California, I fed our homemade RATG into the fluid flowing directly into Jim's veins. Jim remembered all too vividly the excruciating pain and debilitating soreness caused by the muscular injections ten years earlier. When I told him we now could give it to him painlessly, a big, broad grin shot across his face.

"Hallelujah," he said. "I hated that rabbit stuff the last time. I still have nightmares about it. It's one of those things that made me think twice about going through this again."

Not until the second postoperative day, after we were sure the bleeding had stopped, did the surgical residents pull out the two chest tubes draining the cavity around Jim's new heart. The process hurt. As they jerked out the tubes, they had to snug down the sutures that closed and sealed the tiny skin incisions in his chest, and the sutures pinched. But Jim much preferred this slight, brief discomfort on the outside to the thought of having the huge tubes sticking up inside his chest.

That day, too, Jim began taking his cyclosporine. When researchers in Cambridge, England, had first tested cyclosporine on rats, they dissolved it in alcohol and injected it. A lot of rats died from renal failure, partly from the alcohol, partly because the drug was toxic to the kidneys. Looking for something else to serve as a base and another way to administer the drug, they made the rats drink it after they had dissolved it in olive oil. They chose olive oil because one of them was Greek and had managed to strike a deal with a local Greek restaurant to supply the lab with whiskey bottles full of the stuff. Though the rats with transplants still had kidney trouble, they began to survive in large numbers and suffered rejection much less frequently. Ever since, cyclosporine has come in an oil base. It is not really palatable. Most patients combine it with chocolate milk.

But Jim hated chocolate milk. So we mixed it into orange juice for him. We could not use the standard hospital Styrofoam coffee cups because the cyclosporine would adhere to the wall of the cup instead of dissolving. So twice each day, once in the morning, once at night, the nurses would pull out the bottle of cyclosporine, accurately measure a dose with a stopper into a glass of orange juice, and hand it over to Jim. Later, he would do the same thing himself, or Shirley would, doling it out in a vital daily ritual.

Before the operation, Jim's kidneys had not functioned normally because his old heart had not been powerful enough to pump sufficient blood to keep them healthy. Moreover, he had been on cyclosporine for so long that he had probably suffered some kidney damage, the most devastating side effect of this wonder drug. The heart-lung pump used during the operation could also cause temporary damage to the kidneys, in part because of lower perfusion pressure during the surgery. Jim's kidneys, helped along by the dopamine and the powerful and effective new heart, had repaired themselves by the third day after the operation, and we could then safely increase the cyclosporine dosage.

By then, we had begun giving Jim the other drugs that, along with the cyclosporine, would make up his three-drug immunosuppressive regimen. Soon after we stopped the massive doses of intravenous steroids, we began giving Jim a much lower dose of prednisone, the only steroid Jim would take regularly—twice a day for the rest of his life. Finally, we gave him Imuran, the brand name for azathioprine, the broad-spectrum immunosuppressant that was the mainstay for heart-transplant patients before cyclosporine.

During his second day in isolation, Jim grew restless.

"When do I get out of here, Doc?" he asked as I checked him over. "And what about something to eat?"

"Tomorrow you can start on soup and liquids."

"Hot dog."

"And I've got you back on Imuran now. I'll give you just enough to get your white blood cell count down to around 5,000, then we'll move you down the hall to the surgical intensive-care unit. Probably tomorrow as well."

"Will I have a window?"

"Yes," I said. "And a television. And Shirley can visit more often. It isn't home, but it's better than this isolation room."

Isolation drove patients batty. Visitation was strictly limited, and everyone who went into the room wore a mask. Before they entered, they had to wash their hands. The masks depersonalized the atmosphere and in truth—although I did not admit it openly—were not all that necessary. But we encouraged them as a way of reminding hospital personnel and visitors that these patients, more than anyone else in the hospital, were vulnerable to infection. Even common germs could kill them, and micro-organisms were ubiquitous, especially in the hospital, where there is so much disease. Germs thrived in hair, on skin, in the creases of a palm. Washing your hands before you entered the room could literally be a matter of life or death. Visitors with the slightest sniffle or softest cough were prohibited.

The costs of such vigilance, however, were psychological and real. For days Jim lay in bed, constantly poked and pounded. He had only the briefest of conversations and saw nothing human but a raised eyebrow or two. He had his new heart, and now he just wanted a television above his bed, a telephone at his side, and Shirley to hold his hand.

We moved him on the third day. We stopped the antibiotics to avoid the emergence of "super bugs." In our quest to prevent infection by using antibiotics such as penicillin, physicians had probably been too liberal. We had overused and thereby abused them, allowing bacteria resistant to the miracle drugs to spawn strains completely unaffected by common medicines.

We also removed from Jim's penis the catheter that drained his bladder.

"That's new," Jim matter-of-factly told the nurse who pulled the tube out.

"What?"

"They didn't use that at Stanford. Not there," he laughed. "They stuck it right through my skin," he said as he pointed to a spot just beneath his naval.

"That's right," I said, looking up from Jim's chart. I realized the nurse didn't have a clue as to what he was saying. Jim was a careful observer.

"Times change, huh Doc?" Jim said.

"You got it. We used to think that thing—it's called a Foley catheter—would cause infections. But we learned from watching guys like you at Stanford that it was no more risky than what they used back then—a so-called suprapubic cystocath."

"Right," Jim said. He grinned at the nurse. "A bladder tube. I hope you learn something this time, too, because I'm not real keen on having this thing stuck up my—"

"We'll conduct a clinical study," I said. "See if we can't get rid of it."

All three of us were laughing, but I was only half joking. In transplantation's infancy we worried that the Foley catheter would provide a perfect passage for lethal bacteria to crawl into the body. Through clinical experience and controlled observation we discovered that the risk of infection from the Foley was actually less than that from the cystocath passing through the abdominal wall directly into the bladder. This was one of a myriad of changes caused by scientific studies of what worked and what didn't. It was a never-ending process. Everything Jim went through now would teach us something about redo transplants, something we could use to help others down the line.

Now that he was in his new room, Jim's spirits seemed high. I thought it might be a good time to tell him about his son.

"Jim, look, there's something we need to talk about."

His smile vanished, I could see him fighting panic as he

looked around the intensive-care unit, then looked out the window.

"What is it?"

"No. No. It has nothing to do with your recovery. You're doing fine. Just perfect. I'm very pleased. It's Jimmy. I'm afraid I can't let him in to see you quite yet. He has a cold, and we'd better not risk it."

The fear in Jim's eyes turned to disappointment as he said, "Whew, I thought something was really wrong."

"I'm sorry," I said.

"I understand. But you'll let him come in as soon as he can, right?"

"You bet. As soon as I think it's safe."

The next morning the physical therapist brought a stationary bicycle into Jim's room so that he could begin the exercise program that would continue well beyond his stay in intensive care, beyond his days in the hospital. Most heart patients have been sick for a long time before their operations. Unable to exercise, their muscles atrophied, their bodies grew thin and weak. As early as possible, we started them working to improve their muscle tone for both physical and—to my mind, more importantly—psychological reasons.

For the most part, the triumphs of postoperative care were invisible to the patients. Changes in the white blood cell count or urine output or blood pressure or heart rate were all plotted hourly on their charts, but the patients never saw this data. Feeling stronger, riding a bicycle for even a short period of time, exercising progressively more each day helped them realize that they were indeed getting well.

We also encouraged transplant patients to become self-sufficient from the outset. For the rest of their lives, they would need to treat themselves much as we had treated them that first week. They would carefully monitor their own temperature and vital signs, adhere to their diet, keep to a regular regimen of exercise, take some fourteen pills a day at exactly prescribed times. Unlike most other patients, they became their own health-care managers, sensitive to their bodies, making crucial decisions about maintaining their health.

On the fifth day after surgery, we stopped all of Jim's intravenous medicines, including the dopamine and Isuprel. We left only two small wires attached through his skin to the surface of his new heart, just in case we needed to pace his heart or alter its rhythm electrically. Removing the catheters, tossing away the IV tubes, throwing out the plastic bags full of sugar water and medicine—Jim's untethering was almost ceremonial. Free of artificial supports, his new heart beating strongly, he now had a new chance at life. That morning, Jan handed him a large calendar marked with the exact times for taking his medicines. His self-care had begun. Symbolically, he was on his own.

Postoperative patients measured their progress in a series of small victories. Six days after his operation, Jim managed his first bowel movement, no insignificant event for post-surgical people. The anesthesia we gave him during the operation had caused his intestines to slow down, then go to sleep for a while. Now they slowly began to awake. Life was returning to normal.

We, on the other hand, measured Jim's progress by a legion of laboratory tests. Once a week during the first three weeks, we ran an extensive battery of blood tests and important surveillance cultures taken from his bodily secretions. The day he moved his bowels, we collected vials of blood, culture swabs from his throat and lungs, and twenty-four hours' worth of urine. We sent them all off to the lab to check for viruses and bacteria, hoping to corner any infections right at the beginning, before they became overwhelmingly difficult to treat, and to make sure that his kidneys and other organs were functioning properly.

The ultimate measure of Jim's progress, however, was how well his new heart fared. And we tested that exactly a week after the operation with Jim's first heart biopsy.

In the old days, when Shumway was still using what is now referred to as conventional immunosuppression—steroids and Imuran—you could tell when a patient was rejecting his new heart by his hemodynamic deterioration. His blood pressure would fall rapidly or his heart rate would change or he would develop an arrhythmia, or irregular heartbeat. But cyclosporine changed all that. It not only prevented most rejection—it made rejection more subtle, more insidious, and thus more difficult to detect.

Phil Caves had only just perfected the biopsy as a way of detecting rejection when Jim had his first transplant in 1976. The technique has since become standard. Every seven days for at least the first three weeks, we performed a heart biopsy. After patients left the hospital, we biopsied them once a month during the first year, then every three months after that. And if we had reason to suspect rejection at any time, if a recipient ran a low-grade fever or showed an irregular heartbeat, if we found anything out of the ordinary, we performed an emergency biopsy. It was the only way we could tell for sure what was happening.

Over the years, Jim had had scores of biopsies. He was a veteran, an expert, a world-class authority on the procedure. Because he had had a bad experience with a biopsy at Vanderbilt months earlier, I was determined to do his biopsies myself.

When the nurses wheeled Jim into the procedure room, I could sense that he was nervous. Jim's obvious anxiety, however, came not from fear of pain or discomfort, which should be minimal when the biopsy is handled properly, but from his understanding of what the results would signify. In a few hours, we would know whether his body had accepted the foreign heart, whether his postoperative course would run as smoothly as it seemed to be running, or whether he would have to suffer through one episode of rejection—or more.

As I cleaned Jim's neck with iodine solution, he chattered on and on to the nurse about how proficient I was at biopsies. I joked with Jim and the nurse, suggesting that I must have given him too much Valium, making him delirious, irrational.

"He doesn't know what he's saying," I said.

He lay there on his back, his head turned sharply to the left, exposing the area I had painted orange. I injected a local anesthetic into the skin on his neck just to the right of his Adam's apple. He had dozens of tiny white scars here from all the other

76

biopsies, crisscrossing lines that spanned the history of transplantation. He was living proof that transplantation worked.

When I was sure his neck was numb enough—I wanted to be positive that he would not feel a thing—I inserted a needle into his jugular vein. I then ran a long, flexible wire through the needle to serve as a stylet. I took the needle out and slipped a eight-inch white sheath that looks like a drinking straw over the wire stylet. The sheath provided easy and secure access to the vein throughout the procedure. Through this sheath I could introduce and remove the biopsy instrument, or bioptome. The bioptome was nothing more than a two-foot long encased wire with two small sharp cups at one end. These cups operate like an alligator's mouth to snip off pieces of muscle from the inside of the heart. The entire procedure would take only fifteen minutes, and it was simple enough that we used only local anesthesia, leaving the patient awake, though occasionally we gave a nervous patient a tranquilizer beforehand.

Once I had the bioptome threaded through the sheath into Jim's jugular vein, we wheeled over the fluoroscope, a small, portable x-ray camera. We positioned it over Jim's chest so that I could follow the bioptome's progress on a television at the foot of the operating table.

Jim's heart appeared on the screen as a vigorously pumping transparent shadow. We could hear the regular, monotonous cadence of the beats on the heart monitor. The lighter shadow of the bioptome snaked into view, and I used the TV image to manipulate the wire down Jim's jugular vein, through his superior vena cava and his right atrium, and into his right ventricle.

Suddenly, we heard loud, irregular beeps as Jim's heart took a few extra beats. The nurse's eyes met mine. Normally, this alarm meant an emergency requiring urgent treatment. Not in a biopsy.

"It's OK," I reassured the nurse. "The bioptome is just tickling the inside of his heart. It will pass in a few seconds."

Watching the screen, I opened the bioptome's jaws and clamped down, biting off a piece of heart muscle the size of a pinhead.

I pulled out the bioptome through the sheath in Jim's neck.

Using a needle, the scrub nurse scraped the tiny piece of tissue from the little cups and dropped it into a jar filled with formalin fixative. Then I repeated the process, snipping off four more tissue specimens. When I was done, I withdrew the sheath and put a Band-Aid over the small incision in Jim's neck. Another battle scar, I thought. I took the five pieces of heart down the hall to Jim Atkinson in the pathology lab as the nurse escorted Jim back to the intensive-care unit.

"How's our boy doing?" Atkinson asked, as he began processing the specimens with his long, lanky moves.

"You tell me," I said. "Everything is right on course in my department. Clinically he's as stable as a rock."

"Well," he said. "I should have good news for you, then, in about four hours."

"I hope so," I said.

When he had finished freezing and cutting the specimens, Atkinson would mount each piece on a glass slide and stain them with a series of red and blue dyes. Each hue would be taken up by a certain type of cell. Then he would slide the little glass mounts holding the minuscule slices of Jim's heart under his microscope and look among the pastel pinks of normal heart muscle for infiltrates of darkly stained inflammatory cells.

If he found any, Jim Hayes was rejecting the heart.

4

Jim Hayes's first week post-op was something of an intellectual treat for me. When I came to Vanderbilt, I adopted the Stanford protocols I had learned during my training, and it was fascinating to listen to Jim's comparisons between his two transplants. Remembering that Shumway had first avoided the Foley catheter or hearing Jim's relief at not having RATG shot directly into his thighs brought home for me how so many of us from Stanford were now running our own programs at different hospitals across the country, modifying what we had learned in California, building on Shumway's work, incorporating our own experiences.

Spending so much time thinking about Jim and his first transplant, I often found myself growing nostalgic for the Stanford years. It was then that I really began to feel good about what I was doing. Before, there had always been nagging doubts. But in California, doing transplantation as Shumway was creating it, I felt all my abilities and talents coming together, the disparate strands of my past and my training and my personality suddenly coalescing.

I had been to Stanford on two occasions several years apart before I finally moved Karyn and Harrison across the country from Boston. I was in college the first time. I flew out to interview for medical school, met Shumway, and was very impressed, especially by his easy manner. Five years later I returned for another interview, this time for the cardiac residency program. I was struck again by the aura of relaxation and cooperation that existed within a program clearly characterized by high quality medicine, discipline, and hard work.

During my two years of thoracic fellowship in Boston, I kept thinking about my impressions of the Stanford program, contrasting the atmosphere there with that at Massachusetts General Hospital, burdened as it was by huge egos and hot tempers and all-too-frequent petty humiliations. When Shumway offered me a year-and-a-half fellowship in transplantation, I jumped at the chance.

For our first six months at Stanford, we leased a home and a car from a professor on sabbatical. The clay-colored stucco house, typically California with a swimming pool and flower garden in the back, lay in the hills behind the main campus, in the Stanford faculty ghetto of large, attractive homes. After the professor returned from his leave, we bought a Volvo station wagon and moved to a newer house in nearby Menlo Park. The place was airy, bright, clean—and expensive for us.

But I had spent the last ten years dragging Karyn around, across the ocean to England and back, living in cramped one- and two-bedroom places off narrow, crowded streets. Now I wanted something better for her. And Karyn loved the new place. So did Harrison. The neighborhood was a delight, and the enclosed backyard lined with brightly colored flowers was heaven. Every night after dinner, on the way back to work, I celebrated those pleasant times with a large chocolate milkshake from Bud's Ice Cream just down the road. I put on weight. So did Karyn. Nine months later, Jonathan joined the happy crew.

I still worked too much, as I had during my seven years of surgical residency at Mass. General, but for the first time since medical school I was able to spend at least five nights a week sleeping in my own bed. At first, the few hours I saw Karyn each night made the time seem like a vacation. If I nevertheless continued to cheat my sons and my wife of the father and husband they had a right to expect, I had a good excuse. My job at Stanford was a dream come true, a once-in-a-lifetime opportunity to learn about the most revolutionary field in modern medicine directly from the most experienced people in the world, from the very doctors who had discovered all knowledge of heart transplantation. It was a rare opportunity, one I had to take advantage of. I devoured it. And I loved the people I worked with.

80

I began not at the busy Stanford Hospital but down the road at the Veterans Administration Hospital, where the pace was slower and I had the opportunity to master the particular techniques developed by Shumway. I learned the Stanford techniques not on transplants but on more routine cardiac surgery, such as coronary-artery bypass surgery and valve replacements. Though the results of those operations were the same no matter what technique was used and the Stanford style was only one of many regional variations, Shumway's methods were so alien to me, so totally unlike those I had learned in Boston, that I felt as if I were learning heart surgery all over again.

In California, for example, we almost always used the electrocautery, a pencil-like device that coagulates blood and burns tissue, to cut and dissect. In Boston we rarely used the device to dissect around the heart, relying on the older technique of sharp dissections with scissors to accomplish the same ends. The technique Stanford used to protect the heart during cardiopulmonary bypass was different and so were a dozen other protocols. I learned that there was certainly more than one way to skin a cat. I enjoyed the contrast and the change, and I exulted in the training.

Two months later I moved over to the Stanford Medical Center and spent four months operating daily with Drs. Shumway, Stinson, and Phil Oyer. During that time, I got my first taste of transplantation. I went on several donor runs. I learned how to harvest the donor heart. The drama, the reversal of a patient's fate, the science of immunosuppression, the challenge of post-op care—I loved it.

The heart staff and residents at Stanford seemed so very different from those in Boston; they did not live in daily fear of their superiors. But the Stanford cardiac surgical residents worked every bit as hard—out of pure devotion and respect and admiration—to please their staff surgeons as did any resident on the East Coast.

In California, the residents in general surgery I worked with were not quite of the same caliber as those I had operated beside at Mass. General. In contrast, the cardiac residents, handpicked by Shumway, were equally as good—probably better. They had spent a long time, a total of three full years, every day and every other night, on the cardiac surgical service.

I was an outsider there. Because I had completed my cardiac residency in Boston, I did not go through the usual three-year cardiac residency program at Stanford. Instead, Shumway had selected me to go straight into transplantation. Yet the other residents, who had every reason in the world to resent my short-cutting intrusion, went out of their way to make me feel welcome.

One, Vaughn Starnes, became my closest friend. Coincidentally, he had done all his earlier surgical residency training at Vanderbilt. Upon my arrival, he took me under his wing. We got along well, understood each other, had similar clinical instincts and standards, and we grew to respect each other both personally and professionally. Although Vaughn was officially my junior resident, he was still teaching me the ropes of the program six months after my arrival. His wife Janet was from Nashville, and it wasn't long before their family of five was spending off hours with our family of four. We had a standing date for lunch, kids and all, each Sunday.

I needed all the tactical help I could get from Vaughn, who had been at Stanford for a year before I arrived. As senior fellow, I was the focal point for the entire heart and heart-lung transplant service. Shumway had devised the program so that a single fellow was responsible for everything that happened in the program. All orders went through him. No medical doctor, no cardiologist, no consultant was allowed to write an order for or even touch a heart-transplant recipient without first checking with the senior fellow. The fellow conducted all rounds. The staff surgeons relied completely on his reports to determine appropriate treatments. He became the sounding board and common denominator for everything that went on with the patients. And he participated in all discussions and all decisions about patient management. Shumway's intent was to insure absolute quality control for these delicate patients—and to train individuals in transplantation like no other program in the world.

My office lay in the Cardiovascular Research Building, a free-standing structure next to the hospital. Barely a year old, the two-story building housed the nonsurgical heart specialists (cardiologists) on one side and the heart surgeons on the other. The building was more or less a tribute to the work of Norman Shumway.

The CRB was very West Coast, laid-back and open, with lots of skylights and manicured gardens. It stood in sharp contrast to those stately, massive, historic Harvard buildings where I first studied medicine. Entering the CRB, one walked past glass windows shielding impressive mainframe computers, which stood guard in front of the huge sun-shot two-story atrium. We conducted all clinical business on the second floor in open offices partitioned off from one another in the middle of the building. The only closed offices, those of the staff surgeons, ran along the perimeter.

Next door, one found more of the same. Built twenty-eight years ago, the Stanford hospital was only three floors high and probably the only hospital in the country with escalators instead of elevators. I was amused by the consensus among hospital personnel that the facility was antiquated and outdated; there was a campaign underway to raise over $100 million for a new facility. My only comparison was the old Bullfinch Building and the Phillips House at Mass. General, where the average room had not been overhauled in sixty years. I knew new from *old*.

Here, palm trees lined the grounds. Hospital staff played tennis outside on long, sunny days. A huge fountain sprayed the pond out front where ducks floated leisurely all summer. Accustomed to the older fourteen-floor hospitals that shot straight up in the middle of a crowded city, where joggers ran to keep warm and motorists would kill for a parking space, I was seduced by the calm, beautiful Palo Alto facilities.

As a newcomer, I couldn't help but notice that every member of the cardiac surgical staff in this medical Eden, except Shumway, wore cowboy boots. What did it mean? Was it some kind of tradition? Some mark of toughness? Were they all hard-core nonconformists? I never did figure it out.

The staff had its share of bizarre personalities. One, not

intimately involved in the transplant program, was simply wild. Brilliant, a technically fine surgeon, he was a workaholic, dedicated to his field, the last to shut down the CRB each night. In addition to the standard-issue cowboy boots, he wore a ten-gallon hat and some way or another knew how to buy plane-loads of ammunition from other countries for his collection of machine guns. A scholar and devoted teacher, he was—let's just say—different.

And then there were the three transplant surgeons, whom I admired and respected each for his own special talents and personality. First, there was Phil Oyer. He spoke in crude and coarse monosyllables, wore cowboy boots of course, rode powerful motorcycles, flew fast airplanes, and held a Ph.D. in biochemistry as well as his M.D. Still unmarried at forty-two, he was my idea of a quietly macho free spirit. He had vast surgical experience, which he could mix with common sense to figure out precisely the right answers to the most perplexing medical questions. He was a skilled Socratic. He could pull from you the exact information you needed to formulate your own opinion, to make your own analysis, to solve for yourself the very problem you had come to ask him about in the first place. It was a tremendous natural talent, one I soon learned to appreciate.

In addition to Phil's interest in cardiac surgery and transplantation, he was fascinated with computers. I constantly found him in his darkened office, his bulky frame lit up by the green glow of his video-display terminal. Until late into the night, he sat there testing, playing, manipulating, and massaging the data in the world's largest transplant database, which he had compiled himself. In addition, he led the clinical development of the Novacor left-ventricular assist device, the experimental electrical artificial heart that will some day have a major role in combating heart failure. He shocked everyone when he finally got married about a month before I left California.

The smartest of the bunch, the man who most inspired me with his technical ability and his intellectual acumen, was Dr. Ed Stinson. Shumway had latched onto Stinson when he was a resident, realizing intuitively that he would make great contributions to cardiac surgery. Shumway sent him off to the National Institutes of Health, the traditional training ground for academic cardiac surgeons, where Stinson would master cardiac physiology and learn everything he could about the field. Since then, Stinson had spent his entire professional life at Shumway's side.

Stinson very quickly became the backbone and the guts of the Stanford transplant program. Shumway encouraged him, inspired him, and gave him room to grow, but as Shumway himself told me many times, without Stinson the program would never have been the success it was. Indeed, transplantation itself would have remained an unrealized dream. Shumway always paid tribute to Stinson as "A man for all seasons, immunologist, infectious disease expert, and cardiac surgeon extraordinaire."

An introspective, withdrawn island of a man, Stinson avoided national meetings and forums. Thin, birdlike, his black hair combed straight back, Stinson focused on his research and the clinical developments at Stanford. Sometimes ill at ease in crowds, Stinson loved the simple life, spending a month every year working on his ranch in northern California. He was the type who might not ever make it in private practice—where excessive back slapping with referring physicians is de rigueur—because of his shyness. But he was in a class by himself when he was working out of the public eye with like-minded colleagues on tough problems.

Stinson approached the entire field of cardiac surgery systematically, clearly defining the important problems in his own mind, then designing clinical studies and basic scientific research to solve those problems. His absolute intellectual honesty explained his ability to ask just the right questions. His stubbornness and persistence in asking those questions again and again until they were answered accounted in large measure for the Stanford program's string of accomplishments. Breaking down the seemingly insurmountable challenge of transplantation into many small problems, he conquered them one by one.

If Stinson was the mastermind behind transplantation,

Shumway was the inspirational leader, the guiding spirit who pulled it all together with his vision, his determination, his unrelenting commitment, and his dedication to those who worked for him.

A playful spirit, Shumway had an almost pathological love for one-liners. Whether he was charming nurses, disarming his critics, or trying to teach you something profound in a painless way, he always had a new joke.

If the jokes were sometimes risqué, he handled it all with aplomb, even with a peculiar kind of dignity and grace. A master juggler and magician, he was the best face a transplant program had ever put toward the world at large.

He was a great surgeon but an even better teacher. Calling himself "the world's greatest first assistant," he could march a resident painlessly through the most challenging cases. He was always out to make those around him look good, including the green, fumbling residents he was trying to teach. "Never be afraid to double dribble," he would say, working across the table from you, making sure you took two separate deliberate passes with the needle in a tight spot in an anastomosis, rather than flamboyantly trying—with more speed but less care—to take it all in a single swoop. He kept the pace of the operation moving, using positive reinforcement, telling you "that's a good stitch" even when you knew it was awful. More often than not, you made sure the next one was perfect. He made you want to please him, not out of fear, but out of respect. You admired him.

"Cardiac surgery is not hard to do," he would tell his young residents. "It's just hard to get to do." And they would learn what he meant, putting up with years and years of apprenticeship, of watching operations, of falling asleep in the OR while holding a retractor after a long night without sleep. Four years of college, four of medical school, at least five of general surgery spent living in the hospital, a year or two of research, three of cardiothoracic surgery—it was a long haul, but residents came to the transplant program yearning for challenging work on one of medicine's frontiers.

When they got there, Shumway insisted that they keep their operations, their brutal manipulations of the human body, as simple as possible. Some surgeons made heart surgery so complicated that it was confusing, and Shumway believed that urge was the cause of most unsuccessful cardiac operations. "Keep it simple," he'd say over and over. "The simpler it is, the less room there is for error. If it looks complex, it's not right."

Shumway was one of a kind, but he was also human. He could be irritatingly hidebound. For example, he refused to use cardioplegia, the solution we injected into the aorta to stop the heartbeat suddenly and to keep the heart asleep and motionless for the hour and a half it might take to fix it. Over the last decade, respected researchers and scientists had published thousands of papers, indeed had made their whole careers justifying their claims that cardioplegia was essential to the safe conduct of heart operations. Shumway knew better. He did not believe them, and he told them so publicly. He preferred to protect the heart more simply. He poured ice-cold saline over the heart throughout the operation, slowing its metabolic rate. He laughed at those who spent their lives dwelling on a solution he felt was unnecessary for most heart cases. He may or may not have been right, but it was hard to argue with his results, which were as good as or better than others obtained with cardioplegia.

During my years at Stanford, Shumway only occasionally participated directly in the transplant operations. Having spent long and hard years in the laboratory working out the surgical techniques and therapeutic care, he now relied principally on his associate surgical staff and cardiac fellows to run the program. But he was there at each and every Friday-morning transplant conference, and he kept his finger on the pulse of the place. His word was still law, and he roamed the program, immediately taking up any problem that interested him, for all the world like a kid opening presents at Christmas.

He relied heavily, too, on his nurses—a habit I admired and somewhat adopted at Vanderbilt. He made rounds with them, telling his jokes, always keeping them on their toes with his funny but penetrating questions, always upbeat, always enthusiastic, but never holding back any punches. If they'd made a mistake, they knew it. But they didn't hate him for telling them, they didn't walk about suppressing some smoldering resentment. Unlike many surgeons, Shumway never made them feel as if the mistakes came from a defect in their characters. Once, after he had referred to his nurses as his "colleagues" in a scientific paper, they responded with a birthday cake topped by one word: COLLEAGUE.

Shumway got away with his jokes and his quirks because, more than anybody else in the world, he had a feel for transplantation, a sixth sense for making good decisions and finding the right answers. An uncanny judge of people, he could pick out immediately those who handled stress well, those who could function in top form in tight situations, those who knew how to deal with their personal feelings, those with the character and the personalities to be great surgeons. It was, I think, his most valuable asset, this ability to size up an individual, to know who would be a winner, who would make the important contributions to cardiac surgery.

Not surprisingly, he attracted such people. He encouraged them. He inspired them. He tolerated and never discouraged their eccentricities, brought their creative potential to fruition, trained them in his unique tradition, and then sent them on their way to become leaders in the field. In a profession filled with cutthroat ambition and big egos, he knew how to be a father. He peopled the hospitals of America, coast to coast, with his talented and proud surgical students and surrogate sons.

"The six months you spend running the transplant service," Stinson had said when I first arrived at Stanford, "will be the most powerful six months of your life." And he was right. Under the impress of their personalities, their technical skill and experimental passion, I emerged from the Stanford experience so deeply involved in the world of transplantation that I knew I would never shake free.

My transition to senior fellow in transplantation led me straight to the center of this brave new world. When I had been a chief resident, I had a team of junior residents working under my command. Now, it was just me. I handled the scut jobs that interns, some seven years behind me in training, would have handled elsewhere. I did the diagnostic lumbar punctures, inserting needles into the spinal columns of fever-ridden patients. I drew the blood cultures. I changed the central venous lines and the arterial catheters. I even changed the dressings when necessary. No job was too mundane.

Shumway felt you could learn transplantation only by total and absolute immersion. Nobody looked in. No one was around. If I wanted to know something, I had to set up the consultation. It was a tremendous responsibility accompanied by a good deal of stress. I was under fire. I learned quickly not to miss any details and to settle for nothing less than perfection. I had to move fast to diagnose infection or rejection, because if I didn't, the patient would die. Missed details cost transplant patients their lives, more so than in any other branch of medicine.

I came out of Stanford knowing how to care for the sick, how to assess difficult clinical situations, how to move quickly and efficiently, how to work with all support people, including—and especially—the nurses. I learned how to make the people around me trust me and have faith in me, to feel good about the work they did, to open up, to give me the right information unhesitatingly when I needed it. In short, I think, I hope, I learned how to be a leader.

At the same time, the social and ethical issues of transplantation took on a rich fascination for me. They filled a need I had felt ever since my undergraduate days at Princeton when I had entered the Woodrow Wilson School of Public and International Affairs looking for some perspective on my narrow, somewhat privileged, Southern upbringing in a family full of doctors. I felt my interests and talents coalescing in the multidimensional world of transplantation.

I had found my calling.

*   *   *

Even today when I have an occasional difficult case or I feel uneasy about a certain transplant, I will phone Ed Stinson in California. He can listen to all the data I give him and immediately ask just the right question. I thought of calling him to talk about Jim, not because the case was particularly troublesome or complicated, but because of Jim's history, because of his tie with Stanford and the pioneering days of transplantation, because of the continuity. But I wasn't sure Ed would understand my sentiments, and I put it out of my mind.

I resisted the urge to touch base with Stinson even after Jim Atkinson called me to tell me that he had discouraging news. Jim Hayes was suffering from severe acute rejection. The diagnosis concerned me, but not greatly. Perhaps ten percent of patients show some rejection on the first biopsy. Because Jim was a re-transplant, I was a bit more worried than I normally would have been, but to tell the truth, I was more bothered by what Jim's psychological reaction might be.

I would treat him with one gram a day of a steroid called Solu-Medrol for three days running. The treatment almost always worked. Then I would follow up with a biopsy in seven days. Meanwhile, I would tell Jim that—even though the biopsy showed some rejection—there was nothing really to worry about. In fact, I would say, "So far, so good."

I had no way of knowing then, nor any reason to suspect, that Jim was in for much, much worse, and that before long I would indeed be picking up the telephone and dialing Ed Stinson's number.

Part Three

HARD CHOICES

1

Traffic lay thick along West End Avenue, though it was nearly eleven at night. Who were all these people? The bumper sticker plastered across the back of my old BMW said California Transplant. Walter had given it to me as a joke, for in truth I was a Nashville native. Like all natives, I wondered at what had become of my town, how it had grown so quickly, how its very look was changing.

I had just finished rounds and was on my way home when I decided to drop by my parents' place on Bowling Avenue for a few minutes. One thing I knew for sure—the house I grew up in would always be the same, big and white and *permanent*. Dad had meant it to be that way. He valued family above all else, and years ago he stretched well beyond his means to find a home for his wife and five children that would serve as a haven during our childhood and as a retreat when we grew older.

I had reached the end of a hard day and a long week, and I wanted to unwind a bit with Dad and cheer up Mom, whose usual frantic pace had been slowed down by a recent neck operation. It was late, but my parents were used to these visits at odd hours.

The news about Jim Hayes had not been what I had hoped, but I did not feel overly concerned. Both Jim and Shirley seemed to take the results of his biopsy in stride. Not that Jim's reaction surprised me all that much, old pro that he was. Still, his inner strength and optimistic outlook helped to quell any lingering doubts I might have had about retransplanting him. His desire to live life to its fullest was as strong as ever.

I was more concerned with Jean Lefkowitz, a young woman who six months ago had been our first heart-lung transplant recipient. Earlier in the week she had returned to Vanderbilt from Florida, where she had been living with her two young children and her mother, Virginia, her faithful support throughout. To all appearances, Jean had been doing very well in her new life. Suddenly, a few days ago, she developed a serious infection in her transplanted lungs. I immediately had her flown back to Vanderbilt for treatment.

Heart-lung transplants were still quite rare, and we had a lot to learn about the postoperative course. Fewer than a hundred of these operations had been performed worldwide. I had participated in a number of those operations at Stanford, where the first one was done in 1981.

I had planned to offer heart-lung transplants at Vanderbilt from the moment I arrived almost a year before, but it had taken me six months to get into position to do the operation. The team we had assembled was working together well by then, with some ten heart transplants behind it, all the patients alive and well. Heart-lung transplantation, I thought, would not only save desperate people's lives, but would also give a big boost to the program I was trying to build. Vanderbilt would be one of the handful of centers in the country capable of doing the procedure.

Dr. James Loyd, one of the pulmonary specialists at Vanderbilt, had been following a number of patients with primary pulmonary hypertension, a progressively destructive, unrelenting, and irreversible disease of high blood pressure in the lungs. We did not know the cause of this mysterious illness, most common among young women, which affected both the lungs and—secondarily—the heart, but we knew it inevitably led to a premature death. Outside of a transplant, there was no effective medical treatment.

Around Thanksgiving, I told Jim Loyd I thought we were ready to begin doing heart-lungs, and he wrote to two of the patients he had been tracking. He informed them that Vanderbilt now offered heart-lung transplantation, but that it was still generally considered an experimental procedure because so few had been done. Jean Lefkowitz was one of the patients he contacted.

I did not recognize her name when she first called my office. In fact, I was in the operating room at the time, and I misunderstood the message she left. I thought she was after general information about the program we were planning, and I decided to return her call after I got back from a conference on transplantation in Chicago.

I phoned Jan Muirhead the next day from Chicago, as I did daily when I was out of town, to check on the status of my patients and to consult on their treatment. She said that Jean Lefkowitz had called three times since I left.

"Dr. Frist, she's not just after information. She wants us to take her as a patient," Jan said.

I called Jean immediately from the hotel. She quickly reviewed for me her entire medical history and told me something about her family relationships and her financial situation. I explained to her that while we had done a number of heart-lung transplants at Stanford, we had yet to perform one at Vanderbilt. But we were about to begin our program, I said. She said that she was being considered at Pittsburgh, but that she would rather come closer to home in Nashville if possible. She struck me as articulate, enthusiastic, and sincere, and I told her I would be happy to interview and examine her.

At the beginning of December, Virginia Landess wheeled her daughter into my office. A beautiful young woman with quite a head on her shoulders, Jean hardly looked ill as long as she stayed in her wheelchair. But when she tried to walk across the room, she gasped for air, and her true condition became apparent. As I explained all she would have to face, I discovered that she had carefully investigated the field of heart-lung transplantation.

I again emphasized that we were just beginning the program, that the procedure itself was still considered experimental, and that the long-term success rate was not nearly as good for heart-lung transplants as it was for hearts. I told her that in the late

1980s we were where heart transplantation was in the late 1960s. We simply did not know the long-term prognosis of transplanted lungs. On the other hand, the alternative was death. And the survival rate for the operation was comparable to the heart-transplant procedure at a similar stage in its development. The rate was rising as we did more of the operations, learning from each one just as Shumway had learned from each of his early heart transplants.

We talked for a while about Pittsburgh and the fact that she could not raise the $125,000 that the hospital required up front. I told her the money would not be an obstacle for us, though I did not go into the details.

Vanderbilt had agreed when I was hired to accept a handful of indigent patients. This was partly in order to help me build an effective program and partly to improve the hospital's relations with the Nashville community, whose ire had been aroused two years before when Vanderbilt was accused of refusing to accept a penniless burn victim.

During the early years at Stanford, the university had operated its heart transplant program under a federal grant; this enabled the program to take patients on the basis of need, rather than on their ability to pay. But when grant monies ran out, patients without insurance had to put up as much as $100,000 in cash just to be allowed on the waiting list. Hospitals simply could not afford to take such losses, and most insurance companies at the time tagged this new procedure experimental and did not cover these rarer transplants.

The question of finances, of who pays and when, was another of the big social and ethical issues confronting the transplant field. I knew that one day, my honeymoon at Vanderbilt would be over, and my program would have to pay its own way. But for now I was free to re-create the glory days at Stanford. For now, I could help a Jean Lefkowitz if I decided she was a good candidate for treatment.

Jean was staring at me, looking directly into my eyes. She paused. She said, "Dr. Frist, I am very ill. I have two children I

96

want to see grow up. I have been considered by Pittsburgh, and they think I am a good candidate. But I can't come up with the kind of money they want, not in the time I've got left anyway. I have raised some money from bake sales. I've made appeals to the newspapers. I've written to hundreds of businesses asking for money. I've asked everyone to help. I've looked into other programs, like the one in Arizona, but they've done so few. Stanford is just too far away for me, and the waiting list is too long. I'll die before they get to me.

"You were at Stanford. You know how to do the operation. You don't have a waiting list. You're not asking for cash up front. I want to come to Vanderbilt. I want you to do the operation."

And I knew then I would do just that.

She was young. She was confident. She trusted us. She understood our situation. She had a strong will to live. She was ideal, and I was determined to list her.

Because she would be our first heart-lung case, I felt that she should meet with Jim Loyd, with Walter and Jan, and with Dr. Harvey Bender, head of thoracic surgery at Vanderbilt—and my boss. I would be discussing her case with all of them before we put her on the waiting list. Walter was out of town, but later that day Jean saw Dr. Loyd, who agreed that she was a good candidate. Afterward, we dropped in on Harvey Bender, and the chemistry between the three of us seemed perfect.

Jean left the next day for Florida. A week later I called her to say we had accepted her as our first heart-lung candidate. I warned her that we would not be ready to begin the program for another month or so; I needed time to perfect the protocols at Vanderbilt and to train the various people at the hospital. And even then, after we could list her, the difficulties in finding a suitable donor, even harder for heart-lungs than for hearts, might mean a wait of several months. The race between certain death, growing closer day by day, and the nerve-wracking wait for a donor was set into motion.

"I understand," she said soberly, but I could hear the sigh of relief behind her carefully controlled voice.

I spoke with her physician, a Dr. McDonald, who rushed to assure me that Jean did indeed have that invaluable intangible asset, the hard-headed optimism and faith it took to weather the transplant's arduous postoperative course. I arranged transportation for Jean with a company in Florida that had volunteered to fly her to Nashville in their chartered jet at a moment's notice. And then I sent Bob Lee, one of our surgical residents, to look for a couple of sheep I could use to demonstrate the operation.

Around Christmas, we had our dry run. Bob prepped the sheep, and I walked the team of physicians, nurses, and technicians through the excision of the donor heart and lungs from one sheep and implantation into another. I emphasized the important aspects and common pitfalls as I went along: minimize dissection around the trachea, carefully avoid damage to the phrenic nerves in the dissection, spend at least thirty minutes drying up the field before sewing in the specimen, minimize manipulation of the fragile lungs. These were the tricks I had picked up at Stanford, some of which had been learned at great expense early in the development of the procedure.

Walter and I completed the operation as the entire surgical team, including the scrub nurses, circulating nurses, anesthesiologists, and perfusionists, stood around us carefully observing and taking notes.

After the operation, I adapted the Stanford protocols to our situation at Vanderbilt and distributed them to all of the staff who might conceivably become involved in heart-lung transplants. I had urged Bob Lee to find a freezer for storing the preservative fluids we used to protect the excised heart and lungs, mainly because Shumway had always insisted on the importance of the coldness of these fluids, and I wanted a symbol to stress our commitment to the Stanford way of doing things. We found a huge freezer at the supply house, much larger than the one we used in California, and it looked like a giant, alien creature from a Japanese horror movie among the other equipment in the OR. It was a strange tribute to Shumway's influence, but it made the point well enough. Finally, I felt that everyone was familiar enough with the standard procedure, and around New Year's Day I entered Jean Lefkowitz's name on our list.

Now there was nothing to do but wait. Jean Lefkowitz waited for a new chance at life, her only chance. We waited for an opportunity to demonstrate Vanderbilt's expertise as a world-class transplant center, to expand our lifesaving program so that we could help hundreds of other Jean Lefkowitzes and Jim Hayeses. Like the others on the transplant team, like a number of Vanderbilt doctors and administrators, I was excited and a little anxious. For the first time, I think, I felt that odd twinge of conscience I had tried so often to discourage in my pretransplant patients. It hit me that we were waiting for, even anticipating, the sudden death of someone we did not know.

Before the month was out, Jean took a turn for the worse, and she lingered very near death. Twenty-four days after I had listed Jean, a teenage girl in Nashville shot herself in the head. She was brought into Vanderbilt Hospital, where doctors examined her fatal gunshot wound and pronounced her brain dead. Luke Skelley, director of the organ-procurement agency that served Nashville and middle Tennessee, called me at home a few hours later as I sat talking to Karyn.

He told me about the tragedy. He said he had talked to the young girl's mother and received permission to use the heart and lungs. He had run all the tests, and the donor was a suitable match for Jean, having the same blood type and a comparable chest size. He had gone back to his office and processed the information through the national computer network, though by then there was little doubt in his mind that we would pop up first on the list. He grew enthusiastic as he told me everything was a go. We were ready to perform the country's one-hundredth heart-lung transplant, the first ever in Tennessee. Turning away from Karyn's searching eyes, I felt the excitement as well.

I rushed back to the hospital. The heart-lung operation itself was more complicated than a heart transplant. The dissection was much more extensive, requiring removal of all the organs from just below the neck all the way down to the diaphragm, the broad muscle that separates the contents of the belly from the chest. The sight of the huge chest cavity, entirely empty before the implantation of the new donor heart and lungs, gives even the most experienced surgeon pause. The procedure took many more hours, but we were helped both by the fact that we did not have to transport the organs over a long distance and by our months of careful preparation. The operation went off without a hitch, and early the next morning Jean Lefkowitz was on her way to the ICU and her new life, while I sat in the waiting room talking to her much-relieved mother.

It must have been about the time that I walked back to my office that the morning edition of the *Tennessean* hit the stands. I had no inkling of the storm brewing around me when my secretary Faye announced a call from a woman whose name I did not recognize.

Faye said, "You'd better take it. She seems very upset. Something to do with Jean Lefkowitz."

I said, "This is Dr. Frist."

And the voice said, "You heartless person."

She was crying, fighting to talk amid heaves and sobs, her voice racked with anger and pain. She said, "I hope you are satisfied." She said, "You lied to us." She said, "No one was supposed to know." She said, "You promised no one would know." She said, "Are you happy, now? Do you feel good about what you did?" She said, "Oh, you're famous, very, very famous." She said, "But what about my little girl?"

And she said a lot of other things, though none of it made much sense until Jan marched into my office and slapped down the newspaper in front of me. When I saw Jan's face I thought, Something has happened. Something terrible. Jan was clearly upset, not saying a word, and at first I thought that she, too, was angry with me, like the woman on the phone. Then I saw the article, which identified the donor by name, age, and address and described the mode of suicide. The words struck me like punches in the belly.

I was talking to the mother of the young girl who had killed herself the night before.

Somehow, I made it through that conversation. And somehow I made it through the rest of that day. Angry phone calls burned the wires back and forth between the hospital and the newspaper. The press justified focusing on the donor's death by the public's right to know. But did they realize that such publicity discouraged organ donation, tainted our efforts to educate others? Did they realize that they were in effect denying lifesaving opportunity for others waiting to receive hearts? Did they realize that they contributed to the eventual death of these potential recipients? I almost blew up myself when I found out that someone within the hospital staff had leaked the name of the donor and the facts surrounding her death to the paper. But then I noticed that everybody from the nurses to Faye appeared to be in shock, seemed to feel as if they had personally betrayed the dead teenager's tormented mother, as if they were somehow to blame for allowing the unnecessary publicity to intrude on the family's grief.

A pall settled over the hospital. It shook me more than the headlines had. I realized that at all costs we had to make sure that none of this affected Jean Lefkowitz. I told the staff that she must hear as little as possible about what had happened—nothing at all if we could manage it. If we couldn't, we had to make sure that Jean never learned the effect her operation had on the rest of us.

I suppose that I was practicing what a politician might call spin control. But it worked. Instead of fretting over the tragic leak and its deplorable effect on the donor family, members of the transplant team focused on limiting the damage it could do to Jean's post-op course. In short order, we had our priorities back where they should be. Jean became the program's favorite, a brave young woman that everyone was pulling for.

Jean's recovery was not complicated by the story, nor was it unduly complicated by medical problems. But it was difficult. Jan spent many hours helping Jean; she grew extremely close to her patient, now her friend.

At the time, I did not fret much about their rapport, viewing it in part as evidence of my success at damage control. But now, six months after the operation, with Jean back in the hospital, I felt differently. She was very sick. I was afraid she was not going to make it. Each time I saw her that week, I feared it would be the last. And I worried about the effect the death of this popular patient might have on members of the transplant team, especially on Jan.

2

Partly because of Jean, no doubt, I had been thinking a lot that week about publicity. The dead had a right to privacy, and so did their families. Transplant programs and organ-procurement agencies must not only respect this right but guarantee it. The kind of publicity Jean's case had received would strike any grieving family, shocked by sudden death, as nasty and unnecessary.

But the *Tennessean* editors and reporters argued that their readers were interested in transplantation and the many dramatic issues surrounding it—all the issues, no matter how painful. They had a right under the First Amendment to run the story and a real reason for doing so. And, in part, I tended to agree.

Public interest in transplants had been running high since the early 1980s. This was one reason we had seen politicians, even the president, making impassioned and sensational pleas for donor organs and funds for individual patients. The patients themselves, uninsured in many cases, often used the media to raise funds for transplant operations; the transplant literature we handed to patients encouraged this practice as perfectly legitimate. Hospitals depended on good relations with the public they served. They had an obligation to let those in the surrounding communities know that transplantation was available, that it was a viable therapy. And, as competitive businesses, they needed to market their cutting-edge technology and quality care. For all these reasons, hospitals had a legitimate interest in the press covering their new transplant programs.

From my point of view, the more the public heard about transplantation, the more people would come to understand the critical shortage of organs. In the long run, that might help relieve the shortage, save more lives, and make my job much easier. I believed in transplantation, I had seen it work, and I had a positive story to tell. So I kept an open mind, and an open door, when it came to reporters, writers, and the media.

Some of my colleagues, many even at Vanderbilt, frowned on this attitude and accused me of chasing headlines. I knew, too, that for all our vigilance, the names of donors would occasionally be uncovered by an always-aggressive press. But I also felt that as long as we did everything in our power to protect the donor families, it was worth the risk of being called a glory hound to get my life-or-death message across.

And getting my message across also took a lot of simple, hard work. I traveled with members of the transplant team or with Luke Skelley or other coordinators to tiny hospitals around the state, to women's groups, to civic organizations, to high schools, anywhere that would have me, whenever time permitted. I discussed the shortage of organs and the miracle of transplantation. I tried to let people know that there were things they could do. They could realize that transplantation works, discuss their feelings about donation with their families, make their intentions clear to their loved ones, and sign the donor card on the back of their driver's licenses.

I wanted people to know about chimeras like Mark Johnson, who in many ways was an ideal transplant patient. Twenty-one years old, newly married, a passionate deer hunter, at two weeks post-op Mark was going down to rehab every day. He exercised for an hour, cheerfully anticipating his return to work at his family's mattress business and a trip into the wilds of east Tennessee when the hunting season opened. By the time he was six months out of the hospital, he was not only working and hunting deer, but exercising vigorously and occasionally traveling with me to talks and interviews. His rustic good health put to rest any misconceptions audiences had about transplant recipients being helpless invalids.

But he had been an invalid and a very sick man—*before* his transplant. His heart trouble had been caused by a virus, and he had about six months to live when we put him on the list. Because immunosuppressive drugs could possibly have an adverse effect on his future children, we had planned a program of artificial insemination for his young wife, banking his sperm before we found a new heart for him. He hadn't suffered rejection after receiving his new heart, his medical insurance had covered the cost of his treatment and medicines, his young wife was devoted to him, and he had every chance of living a long, happy, normal life.

Mark was what transplantation was all about, and the more people saw of him and others like him, the better off we all were.

My guess was, however, that of all my patients, it was not Mark, but little Jonathan Jones that the press would have warmed to the most. He had been only eighteen months old when we transplanted him. He was the son of a single mother who had five other children and who lived in crowded conditions in east Nashville, without a car or a telephone. He was two months post-op and doing great. Each time I saw him and his mother on their visits to the hospital, I felt encouraged about what I did for a living.

Initially, I had my doubts about transplanting him. First, there were the medical problems. At that time only fifteen babies in the world had ever been given heart transplants. Despite extensive lab work, we still knew very little about the long-term prognosis for those infants. I worried, for example, about the side effects the medicines would have on his growth and whether the new heart, without all its nerves attached, would grow along with him. I thought he might have to have another heart later on, like Jim Hayes, and perhaps a third one as well. This problem loomed large in the equation since so many others were dying while they waited for their first new heart.

Baby Jonathan's medical problems were complicated by social issues. I questioned whether Jonathan could get the care he needed for the rest of his life in a home with no father and a mother already overworked looking after her many other active young children. Without an automobile, how would she ever be able to get back and forth to our clinic each week for his regular checkups? And if he missed those checkups, he would die. The finances, too, could be a problem. We could swallow some of the fees and the costs of the operation, but what about the expensive drugs like cyclosporine he would need year in and year out? If she were ever tempted to cut back by the slightest amount, he would reject his heart. And for a while yet, young Jonathan would not be able to express why he felt bad, and she would have to watch vigilantly for evidence of infections; common childhood illnesses could kill him. Because of his small vessels, the biopsies were more difficult, making rejection that much harder to diagnose. And rejection could strike quickly, almost overnight. With no telephone, Jonathan's mother would not be able to reach us quickly in an emergency.

Finally, there were the psychological effects that walking this medical tightrope would have on Jonathan, his mother, and his brothers and sisters, effects that we would know nothing about for years to come. Jonathan himself could not give his consent to the operation. Should his mother and I force a life on him filled with a certain amount of discomfort and constant anxiety, a life characterized by rigid schedules and severe limitations, by fragility, even estrangement? In twenty years, would he thank us?

Such worries had led most transplant centers to become highly selective in choosing patients, calling for money up front and picking only those who had the best chance for a normal life—like Mark Johnson. But that in turn gave transplantation a bad name, a reputation as high-tech treatment for the privileged few, a system of exclusion and limited access.

Ultimately, unknowns of one kind or another defined the entire field, as in any emerging science. They were part and parcel of the transplant surgeon's professional existence.

Also, in the late 1980s, medical knowledge had a half-life of less than five years. By the time Jonathan was old enough to start school, all the assumptions under which we now operated would likely have changed. Jim Hayes was a case in point. Based on what the Stanford team knew in 1976, they gave Jim five years at most to live with his new heart. No one could justifiably predict that the treatment then being developed by Shumway and Stinson would work as well as it did; certainly no one could have foreseen the discovery of cyclosporine.

Transplant research was flourishing. Discoveries were made daily. Each national transplant meeting released a flood of exciting developments. I knew that it was entirely possible we would soon develop new drugs with fewer side effects than cyclosporine or the traditional immunosuppressives, azathioprine and prednisone. Some drugs, at least in laboratory animals, promised to control rejection completely. If the laboratory tests held up, if the government approved the drugs for experimental use on patients in a timely fashion, if the drugs proved as safe for humans as they had for rats, the lives of very young patients like Jonathan Jones could change dramatically within a few years. The unknowns, one by one, would be answered.

Already, I and a group of six others across the country had approval to implant the LVAD, a left-ventricular assist device, as an experimental short-term bridge to transplantation in dire cases. We were working together to improve the device and perfect its use in the lab. There was every reason to hope that one day this modified artificial heart would be as effective for patients dying of heart disease as the artificial kidney had long been for end-stage renal cases. Others were working assiduously on animal grafts, or xenografts. One day, it might be possible to transplant animal hearts into human beings. It sounds far-fetched today, perhaps a bit scary, but it will come. With a little luck, these developments could in a few years help eliminate the donor shortage and free us from the ethical conundrums surrounding the allocation of hearts.

We decided to push ahead with Jonathan's transplant as we observed how totally dedicated his mother was to his future, even in the midst of difficulties I could hardly imagine coping with myself. After all, Jonathan deserved a future alive with possibilities as much as Mark Johnson's as-yet-unborn children and my own three sons. I could live with my doubts, but Jonathan could not live without a new heart.

I was glad now that I had operated, because Jonathan was recovering so splendidly. And transplanting someone like him fit perfectly into the kind of progressive and comprehensive program we were creating at Vanderbilt.

He was also a charmer. About a month earlier, country-music star Barbara Mandrell had gotten in touch with me about the possibility of holding a charity event to publicize and raise money for transplantation. She had a close friend and other acquaintances who needed liver and kidney transplants, so she already knew something about the issues. I was struck by her sincerity and her commitment to the issue. She commanded an audience I could never hope to reach on my own.

I invited her to visit on a day when we held the follow-up clinic, and she met Jonathan. She immediately fell in love with him. She wanted to hold a celebrity softball game, she said. Invite all the popular stars she knew. Go on every major national talk show, do radio programs, the works, tell the world about transplant patients like Jonathan. I knew, of course, that she was attracted to him for some of the very same reasons that I had almost decided not to give him a new heart.

I was thinking about Jean, and Mark, and Jonathan as I turned up the driveway to my mother and father's house. It was late in the first week after Jim Hayes's transplant. Like all doctors, I found each of my patients special in some way. But it also seemed that each of my patients, even when they were doing well, provided me with medical challenges that were unique—or at least atypical. Even my successes would always underscore the problems that lay at the center of transplantation. I had been drawn to the field by the ironies, attracted by the ethical dilemmas. My specialty brought hope to the hopeless, life to the doomed. It offered me a chance to contribute to an evolving medical science. It challenged me at every level. And I loved it, day in and day out, for its endless complexity.

3

In general, I was feeling better every day about my decision to leave California and return to Nashville after seventeen long years. But because I was obsessed with the transplant program, I found days like the one I'd just gone through harder to take than I should. I had spent much of the afternoon and early evening in the operating room, performing a more or less routine coronary-artery bypass. It was journeyman's work. We take several pieces of large vein from the patient's leg and graft them to the coronary arteries that feed the heart. This lets us bypass blockages of the arteries that lie on the surface of the heart muscle. Some 200,000 such operations are performed each year; they were an essential part of my responsibilities at Vanderbilt.

Heart disease is the number-one killer in America, with upwards of a million people succumbing every year to heart attacks or other cardiovascular ailments—almost as many as to cancer, accidents, pneumonia, influenza, and everything else combined. When any two Americans died, one of them did so from a bad heart or clogged vessels. Fortunately, the death rate from cardiovascular disease was dropping, in part because people had adopted healthier ways of living and diets lower in cholesterol and saturated fats, and in part because of advances in medical treatment. For example, bypass surgery was not even possible before 1966; now it's one of the most common operations.

Transplantation, for all its drama and its high profile, was a treatment of last resort, the place we turned after we had tried everything else—all medicines, dilatation of arteries, even prayer. I had best remember that, I thought. After all, it had been routine bypass surgery that had saved my own father's life fifteen years ago. Without it, I would not have been visiting him now. Without it, Dad would not be standing there, his 6'3" slouching silhouette outlined in the glass front door.

"I heard you pull up," he said, opening the door for me. The gravel in his speech always reminded me how fragile he was. The stroke he had suffered some years back had affected his speech and occasionally made him difficult to understand.

"Were y'all in bed?" I asked, knowing they never turn out the lights until well after eleven o'clock.

"No. No. C'mon in. Mother'd love to see you. We were just talking abut you. About Karyn and the boys."

His voice, barely a whisper, was eerily audible in the still dark night. Every sound seemed magnified, including the slam of the car door behind me. A forceful yet warm and charismatic speaker before the stroke, Dad was frustrated by his crippled speech. His mind was sharp, and despite the whisper he continued to accept invitations to give talks almost daily. He also continued, at age seventy-eight, to put in ten-hour days as the father-figure and ceremonial head of Hospital Corporation of America, the huge hospital firm he had founded with his close friend Jack Massey and my brother Tommy.

Though he never totally regained his fluency, his determination carried him through, as it always had. Nothing stopped him, not the fractured neck he suffered a decade before in a car accident, not the colon cancer he had had removed five years ago, not the heart attack, not the stroke. Wherever he went, his audiences greeted him with respect as the grand old man of American medicine. With his thinning reddish-white hair and his wire-rimmed glasses, he exuded trustworthiness, sincerity, and hope. He looked like a small-town doctor, which at heart he was. The embarrassed shuffle, the humility with which he accepted the accolades and fame he had earned had won the admiration of high-powered New York investment bankers, former patients, fellow doctors, and hospital orderlies. He was a resilient man, an inspiration, but the whisper betrayed him. The whisper carried with it the garbled note of his mortality.

I remembered the first time I heard that whisper, when I

understood that this man, my father, could die. To this day, I have never been so frightened. I was in the middle of my first clinical rotation, my second year of medical school, the time when a student finally gets to treat patients. Two weeks before, Dad had a heart attack and underwent emergency coronary-artery bypass surgery. I flew home from Boston immediately and found him recovering nicely, as I expected, given the fairly routine operation. He gently ordered me back to school. The next weekend, he developed chest pain and coughed up blood. His doctors diagnosed pulmonary emboli, or blood clots in his lungs, which greatly complicated his case. I flew back down. The doctors, Mother, my brothers, all said there was nothing I could do. He would get better each day, but full recovery would take weeks. I should be attending to my studies, they said. That's what he would want. I was torn. I wanted to be with him, but I also realized that my family was right. I returned to Boston, went back to the daily grind, saw patients, followed doctors around, tried to make sense of what I was doing. Five days later, my brother Bobby phoned me from Nashville. Dad had suffered a stroke.

The first morning Dad talked to us after the stroke, I was tired in a way I had never been before, tired not just from the loss of sleep, but from the exhaustion that signals the approach of despair. Then I heard the voice, and I could not understand what he said. That was almost fifteen years ago, but the whisper has been with me ever since. Eventually, Dad stabilized, got better, and resumed his clinical practice, continuing to work with Hospital Corporation all the while. I went back to Harvard and finished medical school. I stuck out my residency at Mass. General. I went on to Stanford. Years before, I had left Nashville for Princeton to prove to myself that I could make something of my life outside the immediate reach of my family's influence. The logic of that initial decision pushed me toward each subsequent one. But every time I talked to Dad, the whisper urged me home.

Now that I was back living in Nashville, it was Mom I was most concerned about. She had always been an outspoken, vigorous, and active woman who enjoyed nothing quite so much as intellectual daring. She read constantly, seemed impatient with the hidebound opinions of many of her acquaintances, and loved to provoke them with her own well-articulated views. I particularly cherished the memory of how she had outraged most of the prominent conservative businessmen around town with her open opposition to our country's involvement in Vietnam in the early 1960s.

I remembered her as selfless, never satisfied unless she was helping others, usually acting behind the scenes. When I was a child, Dad was gone every night, seven days a week, although he always made it home for an hour around suppertime. He had the busiest and largest internal-medicine practice in middle Tennessee, and house calls across the state formed an integral part of his job. That left Mom to carry the load of raising the children.

She thrived on the constant care and attention five growing children demanded. She was always busy, not only looking after us but serving as surrogate mom for half the neighborhood. She was always there, and we—of course—took her for granted. It was hard for me to accept what was happening to her now. She had developed cervical-disc disease, and her debilitating arthritis grew progressively worse. I knew she was frustrated by the limitations her condition imposed, even more discouraged than Dad had been when his stroke hit him. Yet she continued her active existence, lively as ever, never complaining, always trying to do things for others, for Dad, and me, and her grandchildren.

Mother put down a book as I entered her first-floor bedroom.

"Karyn and the boys came by today and brought me a picture Jonathan had drawn at school," she said, pointing in the direction of the nightstand. "She says you haven't been home before midnight all week."

I didn't respond to her reminder. Instead, I asked how she'd been, oohed over Jonathan's picture, and kissed her good night.

I joined Dad in the large den for a while before heading home. He asked me, as he always did, about my work at Vanderbilt, and I brought him up to date on Jim Hayes and Jean Lefkowitz. As we talked, I relaxed in his big reclining chair.

112

I had spent my childhood in this very room. Playing sock football with my sisters and brothers. Breaking a glass table once, and destroying several now-forgotten vases. Here, too, I thought, I had treated my first patient, Scratchy. That's when it all began. The day I cured Jimmy Shapiro's dog.

Playing God, I thought. At first, anyway. Jimmy had brought Scratchy over to see me because I was the son of the well-known Dr. Frist. Scratchy's neck had been cut, somehow, and the dog was in pain. The laceration was open and ugly, about three inches long and still oozing. I had run into this very room, looking next to Dad's chair for the familiar big black bag Dad carried on house calls. Inside the bag, I found a small, flat jar with a screw-top lid. I took the brown powder it contained and spread it over Scratchy's wound. I had no idea what I was doing. I didn't even know what the brown stuff was, much less that it would heal the cut. But I acted confident, like this was something I did every day. To my surprise, the next afternoon the wound was almost healed. How did I do that? I remember thinking at the time. Jimmy Shapiro, eternally grateful to me, swore that I was an absolute genius.

I knew I was no such thing. Mother Nature had done all the work. But the wound looked good, the dog was cured, and Jimmy was thankful. I'll always remember the look on Jimmy's face. It was one of the reasons I had gone into medicine.

Of course it was more complicated than that. You could open the Nashville telephone directory and flip to the name Frist and find the letters MD listed after almost all of them—my oldest brother Tommy, my middle brother Bobby, and even my cousin Johnny, who had moved to Nashville years ago for college. So something else was going on.

And that something was my dad.

Most people now associated Dr. Thomas F. Frist, Sr., synonymously with Hospital Corporation of America. They knew Dad had been the driving force behind Park View, a private hospital that he and seven other Nashville physicians had founded in the 1960s because there were not enough hospital beds for their burgeoning medical practices. The beds that were

available were antiquated. Proprietary hospitals, often an out-
growth of a single physician's practice and therefore more often
than not struggling under financial constraints, had earned a
tarnished reputation in the 1950s. The concept of investor-owned
hospitals, where capital to build new facilities and modernize
outdated ones came from the marketplace, had not yet been
invented. No bank would loan them money, so Dad and sixty-two
friends put up their personal assets, this very house included, for
a million-dollar loan to get their facility started.

Jack Massey, Dad's close personal friend and patient, ran a
successful drug and surgical-supply company that had served
physicians and hospitals in middle Tennessee for years. In fact,
when Dad first came to Vanderbilt, he received his first
stethoscope from Massey. Massey, chairman of the board of the
largest hospital in Nashville at the time, had recently taken control of a little-known fast-food operation called Kentucky Fried
Chicken and built it into the largest fast-food franchise in the
world. Because Park View Hospital, along with two other hospitals that Dad and his associate physicians had been involved with,
became the cornerstone of the HCA empire, folks just naturally
assumed that Dad had been the one to bring the successful entre-
preneur into the picture.

But they were wrong. The impetus to apply the principles that
had been so successful in the fast-food industry to hospitals came
from my brother Tommy. He was a flight surgeon at the time,
having completed a year of surgical training at Vanderbilt, and
he was finishing his stint at Robins Air Force Base in Macon,
Georgia. Away from the grueling internship schedule, he had
some time on his hands to think and plan. He thought about
hospitals, acting autonomously in what was really a cottage industry. He thought about how one might use market capital and
public financing to build new, clean, well-equipped facilities, how
these facilities might join together for mass purchasing and might
share services, creating economies of scale unheard of at the time.
At first he couldn't find anyone who would take him seriously, or
at least seriously enough. Dad, whose real dedication was to

caring for his patients, tried his best to talk Tommy out of his far-fetched schemes. He was clearly disappointed that his first son was leaning more toward business and administration than to the daily care of patients.

Dr. Thomas Frist, Sr., did not want Dr. Thomas Frist, Jr., to turn his back completely on the side of medicine he knew was so fulfilling.

"At least complete your training as a surgeon, and then you can do whatever you want," Dad would say, trying to forestall the inevitable.

Soon, it became clear that Tommy would forge ahead with his wild dreams despite Dad's admonitions. He approached Jack Massey directly, and found the kind of enthusiasm, business experience, and financial backing he needed. An attorney, Henry Hooker, provided the legal expertise. Dragging his feet at first, Dad allowed his own deep-seated entrepreneurial bent to surface and soon jumped on board, adding his experience at founding hospitals and his skill in managing their medical staffs. He also insisted that providing humanitarian and high-quality care in pleasant and efficient surroundings would be the guiding principle of the corporation.

Thus began Hospital Corporation of America, in a series of meetings in that very den. It created a new industry that rapidly revolutionized the way hospitals, for-profit and not-for-profit alike, operated. HCA grew rapidly, maintaining its status as the nation's largest and most productive hospital-management chain for over twenty years, with father and son sitting at the top throughout its phenomenal growth. It was listed on the New York Stock Exchange in 1970 and became the first Exchange company to achieve $1 billion in revenues in its first ten years of operation. And it ultimately grew to over 460 hospitals around the world, with 69,000 beds. Its value at the time of a leveraged buyout in 1989 was $5.5 billion.

Dad worked as hard as anybody to make HCA successful, calling on the incredible number of physicians he knew around the country to bring one small hospital after the other into the

HCA fold. They trusted him because he himself was a small-town physician, accustomed to making house calls and tending to the health needs of others, one who just sort of stumbled into founding a Fortune 500 company.

But Dad's life had not always been so charmed.

Some two-thirds of a century ago, his father was the station master for a railroad in Meridian, Mississippi. When Dad was still a child, my grandfather was hit and seriously injured by a train. He had saved a young woman and her child trapped on the tracks when somebody threw a wrong switch. A few months later, he died from his injuries, receiving the Andrew Carnegie and Woodrow Wilson medals for bravery but leaving behind a number of properties with heavy mortgages. My father was eight years old. His mother barely managed to keep the family house. She opened the big home in the center of town to boarders in order to support herself and her three school-age children.

One of the boarders, a physician, became my father's mentor. He tutored Dad in his studies and hired him to work as an orderly in the surgery clinic he maintained in the town's little hospital. He also encouraged Dad to think about a career in medicine. Dad worked at the clinic through high school; he also mowed lawns and did just about anything else he could find to bring in money. The entrepreneurial seeds were sown. He gave Grandmother a portion of everything he earned each month, but he saved enough to attend college at Southwestern in Memphis, where his brother was already studying to be a minister.

From Memphis, Dad transferred to Ole Miss, where he studied pre-med. He raised his tuition by publishing a football calendar, selling advertising space to the local stores, and running a sort of delivery service. He picked up the trunks of the more affluent students as they arrived at the railroad station in Oxford and carted them by mule-drawn wagon to the dorms.

By the time Dad reached Vanderbilt Medical School in 1931, he had his heart set on becoming a surgeon. Once again, he financed his education with odd jobs. He produced a football desk blotter with advertising all around the edges and the football schedule in the middle. He set up a laundry service for hospital uniforms. He introduced vending machines to Vanderbilt. He even ran a boarding house during the Depression called Paupers' Paradise, earning room and board by finding other students to occupy the house.

He got through his second year of residency at the University of Iowa before his luck ran out. He could not financially afford to continue his residency training, receiving only room and board as compensation. Fortunately, he had already met and fallen in love with Mother.

Dad had skipped a couple of grades and was two years younger than this classmates; though he was four years younger than his brother, Dad was only two years behind him in school. His older brother was a brilliant student and sterling athlete, and my father always felt overshadowed by him. Because he was younger than his friends and because his brother dominated his crowd, Dad had always said he grew incredibly insecure. As a result, he leaned heavily on his mother for a sense of self-worth.

Dad was a straight arrow: he never smoked, drank, or used the Lord's name in vain. He wrote home to his mother every day. He sent her part of everything he earned. But he also felt something was missing in his life, not surprising for a young man who had lost a father suddenly. Though he worked hard and single-mindedly pursued his education, he was nagged by doubts.

But not until he met Dorothy Harrison Cate while at Vanderbilt Medical School did he realize that those doubts also included his intended, his sweetheart from Meridian. She lacked, he realized, what he would one day call warmth. At the time, however, he simply had a vague notion that something was wrong with their relationship. With what must have been some difficulty, he broke it off. He began courting Mother.

She was the younger sister of a prominent Nashville internist who had a solid private practice. When Dr. Cate invited Dad to become his partner, Dad relinquished his dreams of a career in surgery, quit his residency at Iowa, and returned to Nashville sooner than he had planned. He began practicing internal medi-

117

cine, became an Instructor and later Clinical Associate Professor of Medicine at Vanderbilt. He supplemented his limited income as Dr. Cate's assistant by working extra hours at the state penitentiary and by giving routine insurance physicals. And he married Mother.

After spending the years of World War II as a Major and Chief of Internal Medicine at Maxwell Field Air Force Base in Montgomery, Alabama, he returned to Nashville, where he set up his own practice. He began, as had his father before him, to dabble in real estate. The tide had turned for him. Before long his practice was thriving and his reputation as a warm and caring physician and heart specialist was growing. But he never quite shook the insecurities of those earlier years, or so he said. From those experiences grew the genuine humility that has characterized his personality and bearing throughout his professional and business life, a humility that even more than his accomplishments has made him respected and loved and cherished.

His family had suffered because of his father's heroism. I don't think he ever admitted that to himself, but he knew it in his heart and he fought fiercely against any hint in himself of resentment for that act of bravery. Medicine offered him the two things he most needed—a way to ensure that his family was well provided for and a way to validate the selfless generosity that lay behind his father's impulsive sacrifice. Dad fell absolutely in love with the notion of family. And he became a creature so rare I doubt we'll see his likes again—an honestly humble physician.

None of the Frist males could escape such a powerful influence. I'm not sure whether Dad or Mother hoped that all their sons would become doctors, although I'm pretty sure they did not expect us to do so. I know they never asked any of us to study medicine.

Whether they pushed us to become doctors or not, medicine did have its inherent attractions. It seemed a way to help others, to do good while reaping most of the benefits our society can bestow—prestige, power, and wealth. Yet I was also aware that it was a game of control, a game in which you must have others do what you tell them to do—for their own good, naturally. That kind of control can be very seductive for those with strong egos.

Because I am my father's son, because I had the opportunity to see the genuine caring that can and should be central to the practice of medicine, I grew to detest the domineering, demanding, and dismissive doctors that strong egos, longing for a sense of control, could sometimes produce when they were weaned by the brutal rites of passage we called medical training. True, I understood the game almost instinctively the day I cured Scratchy, and I admit it was attractive—to a seven year old.

But that's not why I do what I do. Like I said, I went into medicine because of the look on Jimmy Shapiro's face. That look said that I had made a difference, I had mastered injury and pain, I had become a healer. Every time I remembered that look, I knew how my father felt, knew why he became a doctor. I wanted to feel that way, too. I wanted to be a doctor, too. I wanted to grow up to be just like my dad.

4

When I was a boy, I thought all doctors were like my father, the entire medical profession just an extension of his practice. For me, a doctor traveled about at all hours of the day or night, toting his black bag, meeting and treating as equals people from all walks of life, helping them to get better with kind words, a gentle touch, and the right prescription.

Those images were not entirely a little boy's daydream about his old man. Medical practice did in fact change dramatically over the years. The dominant figure in the profession, the kind of doctor who best symbolized American medicine, used to be the beloved general practitioner, the family doctor who made house calls, understood ordinary people, and gave sage advice not just on health care but on life in general. By the 1960s, he had become the hotshot, highly trained specialist, backed by an arsenal of diagnostic tools and new drugs, separated from his patients by a receptionist, a beeper, and a wall of jargon. When I hit medical school, that figure was epitomized by the cardiac surgeon, the new charismatic breed of doctor, the professional gunslinger dueling directly with death, defeating it with a few sure, deft strokes of his scalpel, then walking off into a fluorescent sunset.

These days the dominant figure was changing yet again. The medical profession had become more complex. Sophisticated technology made health care increasingly expensive. Cures often became corporate ventures, their costs a public issue—rightfully so, with the rapid escalation in price witnessed through the 1980s. In the world of laser beams and computers, diagnosis-related groups, relative-value scales for reimbursement, and health-main-tenance organizations, a doctor needed more than miracle drugs and a steady hand. The hotshot specialists and the gunslingers no longer held center stage. They were being replaced, just as they had once replaced the kindly family practitioner, by the quarterback and his coach, the health care team leader and administrator.

Growing up, the Frist boys were molded by such changes. With Dad a practicing physician, we got an inside view of sorts, and we all responded a bit differently. Tommy became a sort of super administrator, Bobby a busy well-established heart surgeon, cousin Johnny a popular and successful plastic surgeon. I went into transplantation. Even Dad, always searching to create a better environment, demanding quality care for patients, found himself later in his career pulled more and more from direct contact with patients. But he always maintained the perspective of the family doctor, struggling to keep the patient foremost in the minds of those building his hospitals and surrounding themselves with ever more expensive technology. The bottom line, to him, remained the patient.

Now, like benign versions of the Godfather and Michael Corleone, Dad and I would sit in his den late at night, products of two very different medical generations trying to bridge the gap and preserve the best of both. He would say, "Get good people and rely on them," and tell me simple stories of his past when, realizing his own limitations and inadequacies, he had learned to ally himself with those who knew everything he was ignorant of and who could do all he found difficult. I would again describe my transplant team.

"Concentrate on what you have to do with the program there at Vanderbilt," he'd counsel. "Stay away from the tiny hospitals; you don't have the time. Use your talents where they are most valuable. Don't spread yourself so thin." And I would smile, thinking about all the speeches I had made around the state, proselytizing for transplantation and the dire need for physicians to obtain consent for organ donation. I thought about how at each of those little hospitals, someone inevitably would come up after my talk and tell me how, long ago, Dad would drive halfway across the state just to make a house call to a patient in need.

121

And as Michael would say to the old Don, "Don't worry, Dad. I can handle it."

I swear that neither Mother or Dad ever said an unkind word to me. Always, no matter what I did, they were there to back me up. In college and at medical school, when I felt adrift or up against the wall, their letters would arrive saying how proud they were of me, what good common sense I had shown even as a child, how they knew I would excel at whatever I did. Their praise worked. Often, after talking to them or hearing from them, I found myself signing up for a course I had avoided, or taking on a project I had doubted I could pull off, making choices that once frightened me. I could afford to take risks because I knew I always had them. That kind of love, more than anything else, made my background privileged.

When I was younger, it had been Mom who principally protected and nurtured me. Strongly opinionated herself, she understood precisely how to raise children who knew their own minds. She never seemed to challenge their wills. Vladimir Nabokov, the great twentieth-century novelist, wrote somewhere that the worst two words an adult can ever say to a child are *Hurry up*. He would have felt right at home in the enchanted kingdom my mother made of the big white house on Bowling Avenue, where time seemed to stand still and we imagined anything was possible.

There were horses for a while, and later a pool, and a huge backyard. Big brothers to defend me. Big sisters Mary and Dottie to dote on me. The youngest of five children can hardly help but be a demanding little tyrant, and I ruled not just over my family but over my friends—or should I say subjects—who always opted to come to my house to play. No wonder I hated kindergarten and resisted going. My mother's response was to pull me out, take me home, and re-enthrone me.

And when I did venture outside the magic kingdom, Mom worked hard to protect my sense of self-worth. If Woodmont

122

Grammar School conducted a paper drive, she motored me about afternoon after afternoon, making sure I collected more newspapers than anyone else. She helped me sell our raffle tickets to her friends, always buying a few extra herself to give away. When I innocently misled my second-grade teacher about my ability to play the banjo in the upcoming talent show, Mom not only bought me my first toy banjo, but also taught me to play "Home on the Range" respectably enough to get through the show. She wanted me never to know humiliation, never to suffer defeat, never to feel self-doubt. She felt that if she could protect me in that way, I would grow up confident and eventually become independent, strong-willed, a *Frist*.

Even I think she spoiled me. I have long since learned not to apologize for that, but to be thankful instead.

Not surprisingly, with the family emphasis on self-worth, I longed to be first in everything, to be king of the hill, the grammar school *capo di capo*. I imagine I was quite insufferable. I hated—and often too quickly abandoned—anything at which I did not excel. I sought out whatever made me feel useful, different, and in control. I felt most comfortable with slightly younger boys who could look up to me, admire me, the way I admired my brothers and sisters and looked up to Dad and Mother. I found it a virtual sin against nature when one of my young friends, though smaller, could kick a ball farther than I could. I resented anyone my age who was more popular, bigger, faster, or smarter. I was jealous of them. I feared them. They might take over.

The protected little kid became a deadly serious overachiever in high school. The crazy competitiveness and the petty fears, fed by the raging hormones of adolescence, spawned an urge to excel and a desire to lead. At Montgomery Bell Academy, the boys' school I attended, I was elected president of my class three of my four years there. I was editor of the yearbook. I played football. I was voted most likely to succeed during my senior year. I started dating Katie, also a leader at a nearby girls' school and head cheerleader at MBA. I was right on course. I was feeling good about myself.

123

Then I had a motorcycle accident, one that came close to killing me. On a magic carpet ride until then, I suddenly found out that I was mortal. The brush with death punctured my sense of self-importance. The accomplishments I had been so proud of at MBA did not seem tainted so much as they seemed superficial. I questioned to what degree the class presidencies and the accolades of my classmates came as a result of my own talents and abilities, to what degree they came simply as the result of my surname.

Local rich kids, scions of socially prominent families, have few crosses to bear in life, but one of them is that they can never fail, not really, not the way others can. That often leads to envy, a kind of smoldering resentment, even anger, among their peers about their triumphs, but it also diminishes the worth of those victories for themselves. After all, as everyone said, they had all the breaks. Perhaps that's why so many children of wealth self-destruct, throw their lives away on drugs, go wild testing the limits of their own privileges and advantages—a kind of negative challenge, the *only* way they can fail.

That was no answer for me, but I did begin to think seriously about going away to college.

I suppose it's inevitable for an adolescent to feel alienated at some point. In my case, the motorcycle accident gave a romantic patina to an aloofness that had been growing in me since earliest childhood. From the moment I rejected kindergarten, I had been building in earnest what I've come to call the Great Wall between myself and my peers, emotional brick by emotional brick. Only later, however, would I come to believe that every man who wants to lead builds such a wall, though few of them talk about it.

By the time I left for college, the wall was almost complete. Few of my early acquaintances dared or cared to scale it, and I languished behind it without many close friends. I grew more deeply involved with Katie, who knew just where to climb over.

We talked about our lives, our desires, our hopes, our dreams, our plans. Katie, too, wanted a career in medicine, which—since she was the only person outside my family behind the Great Wall—I thought was perfect. We would delay getting married until after we had finished medical school. She would go to Hollins. I would go to Princeton. We would make our marks, then we would join forces, equal and united. It seemed heady stuff when I was seventeen.

Mom and Dad were surprised and a little disappointed at my decision not to stay in Nashville for college. I had never ventured out of the South, nor had any of my brothers or sisters. Why should we? Especially since the motorcycle wreck, my parents worried about losing me. They had imagined that I would stay at home, go to Vanderbilt, and take up medical practice in the natural course of events. Not that they said so openly, but I knew it was the case. I talked it over with my brother Tommy, my guiding light in matters Fristian. He told me to explore the world, go it on my own.

I discovered the Great Wall was portable. I don't mean to imply that I hid behind it, that I was antisocial or withdrawn—in fact, I was just the opposite. I just did not become intimately engaged with others. I kept my distance, I always placed one last emotional barrier between myself and those who would be close. As a consequence, that first year at Princeton was lonely. Dad would write, Mom would call, Tommy would soar up in the planes he had taught me to fly. Those missives, those conversations, those visits were like prison furloughs, human contact behind the wall that made me increasingly value family, like my father before me. And I remained emotionally attached to Katie, my need for her palpable.

I threw myself not only into my studies, but also into student government and extracurricular life. It seemed the more I did, the more I felt in control, the better I liked it. Later, I would worry that I had spread myself too thin, cheated myself of a more emotionally fulfilling college career. At the time, only the ticking off of accomplishments seemed to matter. I became a resident advisor in the dorms, I ran the Big Brother program, I was elected president of the Princeton Flying Club.

By my senior year, I had ticked off enough of them to feel

successful. I was elected vice-president of the senior class, admitted to the Woodrow Wilson School of Public and International Affairs, and I took my medical admissions boards and was accepted to Harvard Medical School. I had spent one summer working for a congressman in Washington, another as an intern at the *Nashville Banner*, mainly writing obituaries. During that last year I had checked myself into a psychiatric hospital in order to write about the civil rights of mental-health patients. Just after graduation, I was elected to the Board of Trustees of Princeton.

During those years, flying—an interest I had adopted from my brother Tommy—grew into a passion. It was the perfect escape, an activity that called for quick decisions and technical mastery, the complete high for a control freak and would-be leader.

I also developed another passion. I was in the midst of a relationship with a dynamic and intelligent woman I had met at Princeton. She had graduated a year before me and had gone to work at the university. She was an actress, active in local theatre, very feminine but with a life of her own, which included a man she had been dating for years and whom she intended to marry.

In the end, I came to love the time I spent at Princeton. As a Woodrow Wilson Scholar I felt in my element for the first time. I was free of formalized study, given full rein to explore issues at my own pace with all the resources of the university at my disposal. I had expanded my horizons, I thought, and handled myself fairly well in the world outside Nashville. And at Princeton, the name Frist might as well have been Smith.

I should have seen my relationship with the woman at Princeton as a warning sign, but I didn't. Instead, I convinced myself that what was wrong between Katie and me was that we were separated, that we needed to be together. After all, I was still under the delusion that I could not make a mistake, that my choices were always right. And I had chosen her.

Katie had said she wanted a career, something to do later on in life when the children were grown, a way to feel good about

126

herself apart from the family. And while that had sounded neat when we were in high school, I realized that it increasingly made no sense to me. Away from home for the first time, I realized how much I idolized my mother and how like my father I had become in valuing the traditional family above all else.

I thought that Mother's selfless devotion to children and mate was one of the highest goals to which a man or woman could aspire. But while my notion of the importance of family had grown stronger over the years, it would be a lie to say that it was the cause of my growing doubts about Katie. It was something else.

Imagining myself as a leader, a Ulysses out on his travels to conquer the world, I possibly wanted a Penelope back home waiting for me and managing the home I so treasured. Or perhaps I did not want to compete professionally with someone who held such emotional power over me. Or it may be that I simply wanted a woman by my side at Harvard to stave off the awful loneliness behind the Great Wall, and Katie couldn't do that if she concentrated on her own career. Maybe all of that was true, but none of it sufficiently explained why I was so uneasy. In truth, I didn't know what I wanted. Tradition had become the convenient mask behind which I was prepared to hide.

I wrote her what seems to me now a caddish letter in which I explained very coldly and calculatedly how I thought her plans to go on to medical school in Texas endangered our relationship and our future. In a parody of my father's passionate faith in family, I argued that what I needed was someone to raise my children and provide me with the kind of emotional support my mother had provided my dad.

She changed her plans. She came to Boston. She went to Boston College, not too far away from the Harvard medical campus. I saw her every weekend. Our relationship survived.

And then there was medical school. Anyone who has been through it will understand; it's almost impossible to describe to anyone who hasn't. It begins insidiously enough with the memorization of mountains of facts, book after book, so much information, so much knowledge, all of it regarded as essential by the neophyte. You can't take it all in no matter how many hours you study. You always fear that if you don't know everything that's dished out, you might not be a good doctor. You might not have the knowledge at hand to take care of patients. You naively try your best to learn it all, to master everything that the young medical student imagines must accompany the trust society places in you when you earn the title of Doctor. From there, slowly over the four years, the laboratory exercises, introductory clinical rotations, and independent study are all piled on in a conscious attempt to guarantee that you don't have time to do things right, that you have to think on your feet, that you have to function well in ever more dire situations when you are ever more tired. It is intentionally rigorous, intentionally threatening, intentionally destructive to your ego and your self-esteem. Or it is at most medical schools.

I came to Harvard starry-eyed and amazed that I had made it there, walking about the ancient and tradition-laden buildings thinking, This is it, knowing that here was where you proved your mettle in medicine. They called Harvard Medical School the best for a reason, and I was here to find out why. Here, I thought, they took the cream of the crop, new and unformed, poured it into a clear and definite mold, and four years later produced the country's leading doctors, who went on to command prestigious medical centers around the world. Somewhere in the middle of it all, exhausted by years of no sleep and high anxiety, doubting every opinion I ever held, questioning every notion about myself that ever kept me going, I realized that instead of molding doctors, medical school was in the business of stripping human beings of everything but the raw, almost insane, ambition you must have simply to get through.

That may be good training for long-distance runners, but I'm not sure it makes for great physicians. Perhaps it works better for basic scientists, who can perform in an isolated world, but a good doctor must be able to respond in a compassionate and understanding way to those around him.

My diary of those years is filled not with talk of high ideals and great aspirations, not even with descriptions of interesting facts I had learned or the fascinating people I had met. There were nutty calculations of how much time I could afford to spend studying for this exam or working on that laboratory exercise, desperate paragraphs trying to schedule some time to sleep, quick questionings of whether time for exercise or food was worth the effort. They were the worries of a young man who had no time to think, who had lost sight of the big picture, who could only concentrate on small things.

Some of the hardening was, of course, necessary. For example, I had always loved animals. My childhood was filled with dogs, hamsters, fish, ducks, cats, horses, even turkeys and alligators. But you could not practice modern medicine without participating in laboratory animal research. Without the sacrifice of rats and cats and dogs and sheep, most of the miraculous things we can do with the human brain and the heart would not be possible. People walking around today leading full, healthy lives would be dead. It was that simple. Humane societies might object, and I would agree if the issue was the humane treatment of animals. But the issue was human lives.

It can even be beautiful and thrilling work, as I discovered that day in the lab when I first saw the wonderful workings of a dog's heart. But the change did not come easy. I came to Harvard the product of a department of public and international affairs at Princeton, an intellectually exciting field that hadn't contributed much to my understanding of the physiology of the liver or the kidneys. I thought I was weak in science and should work especially hard to develop my research skills.

I took six months out of the regular course of study to work in the laboratory of a cardiac physiologist, investigating the effects of hypoxia, or low oxygen tension, on how well the heart relaxes after each squeezing contraction. I spent days and nights on end in the lab, taking the hearts out of cats, dissecting each heart, suspending a strip of tiny muscle that attaches the mitral valve to the inner wall of the cat heart, and recording the effects of various medicines I added to the bath surrounding the muscle.

I was, for the first time in my life, making original discoveries. No one else in the history of man had ever done exactly what I was doing, and I would be able to report my findings to the scientific world in some respected and scholarly journal. The way I acted, you would have thought my project, really very basic, was some grand breakthrough. As I watched the little strip of muscle beat hour after hour through the night in the basement of the hospital, I felt quite pure, as if I were reaching out and touching some eternal truth of nature.

But my experiments were brought to a halt when I lost my supply of cats. I only had six weeks to complete my project before I resumed my clinical rotations. Desperate, obsessed with my work, I visited the various animal shelters in the Boston suburbs, collecting cats, taking them home, treating them as pets for a few days, then carting them off to the lab to die in the interests of science. And medicine. And health care. And treatment of disease. And my project.

It was, of course, a heinous and dishonest thing to do, and I was totally schizoid about the entire matter. By day, I was little Billy Frist, the boy who lived on Bowling Avenue in Nashville and had decided to become a doctor because of his gentle father and a dog named Scratchy. By night, I was Dr. William Harrison Frist, future cardiothoracic surgeon, who was not going to let a few sentiments about cute, furry little creatures stand in the way of his career.

In short, I was going a little crazy.

At one point after my father's stroke, when I actually thought he was dying, I went to visit him in his Nashville hospital room. I actually felt *guilty* about school, worrying that I was falling behind, that I would never be able to catch up. The woman at Princeton and I had parted ways during my first year at Harvard, but before long I became close friends with a fellow medical student. Culturally, we came from different worlds. She was Jewish and liberal. She tried to scale the Great Wall, which was already in danger of collapsing completely under the pressure of medical school and the strain of my relationship with Katie. I had to shore up the wall. I kept my new friend at a distance.

* * *

Something was wrong between Katie and me, but I would not admit that it was us. And it only got worse the first year of my surgical residency at Mass. General. The general-surgery program there was one of the most sought-after residencies in America, and I was determined to do well. I was on call every day and every other night throughout the year, and that took its toll on my relationship with Katie, though I was generally too tired to be aware of what was happening, too occupied and too excited to be depressed.

The subtle and insidious wearing down that had started with medical school continued through residency. Early in my first year, I was one of two interns on the surgical-service team of five residents who supervised the ward care of nonpaying patients.

One night, a seventy-year-old patient developed abdominal pains after a fairly routine chest operation. I performed a careful physical exam of the patient, just the way I was taught, and ordered the standard tests used to help make the diagnosis—a urinalysis, a battery of blood tests, and an abdominal x-ray film. But it was late, I had been on my feet for twenty-four hours, and I had had a hectic night taking care of six other patients, each with their own problems. When all the blood and urine tests proved normal, I called the radiology resident for his interpretation of the x-ray I had ordered. He said it was normal. I did not look it over myself.

The next morning on our five o'clock rounds, the chief resident, seven years and a world of experience my senior, asked about the x-ray. Exhausted from the long night, I muttered that it was normal. He asked to see it. There, clearly shown on the film, was free air in the abdominal cavity, the telltale sign that the patient had a perforated ulcer. The chief resident, in effect my army sergeant, carefully humiliated me in front of my peers, describing my mistake in agonizing detail.

Not long afterward, again on rounds, I reported the results of a urinalysis on a patient admitted with excruciating flank pain, typical of passing a kidney stone. The patient had three or four red blood cells in his urine, but I failed to mention the finding, thinking it insignificant. Once again my chief resident lit into me, intentionally degrading me in front of my fellow residents. I still, today, don't think appearance of the red blood cells was all that important, but I did not know enough then to feel confident in my opinion. I remember vividly the expression on his scolding face and my own sense of shame and ignorance. That was the way we learned to be good doctors.

The chief resident was only following the tradition of the attending staff, which in turn was merely part of the great dictatorial tradition of many, if not most, teaching hospital surgical programs. As I rotated that first year through urology, gynecology, general surgery, and the burn service, I saw the same behavior again and again, training by fear and guilt that at the time I assumed was commonplace and necessary. But I have since come to despise it. Still, all the stress and strain of the constant humiliation did not have nearly so devastating an effect on my psyche as one of my own mistakes.

Fifteen years ago residents and interns had more autonomy in teaching hospitals than they do now. For example, today all emergency rooms are run by specially trained staff physicians who carefully supervise the work of the residents and students. When I was in training at Mass. General, the residents ran both the emergency room and the trauma unit, a practice then common across the country.

I was an intern on the burn service, working under a senior resident two years older than me, when a young eight-year-old girl was referred in from another city. She had burns covering sixty-five percent of her body. My senior resident admitted the patient and the anesthesiologist intubated the little girl, who was having trouble breathing. She stabilized over the next five hours, and the resident went home to get some sleep, leaving me to manage the patients through the night.

About eleven o'clock, I noticed that the girl was clearly having increasing difficulty breathing, and I ordered another chest x-ray and a blood-gas analysis, both standard tests to measure ventilation. The x-ray was crystal clear, but the blood-gas test revealed that the child was very hypoxic, which meant that her body was not receiving enough oxygen. It had been difficult for me to find an artery from which to draw the blood gas because her burns were so bad, and I assumed that explained the low oxygen: I had gotten blood from a vein by mistake.

I repeated the test four times, each time using a little needle called a butterfly to draw out the blood, and each time the blood gas returned the same. The little girl had almost no oxygen in her blood. I didn't know what to do. All appropriate actions had been taken; she was intubated and the ventilator was functioning properly. Her chest x-ray was clear. I was in charge, it was midnight, I remember it was hot, and nobody else was around, so I called the medical chief resident in pediatrics and discussed the situation with him. He dismissed the problem, said that occasionally these young children have low blood gases, and told me not to be too alarmed.

But I knew something was wrong. I sensed it. I didn't know why I was getting the results I was getting, but I should not have been getting them. There was no explanation. I worried about it for almost three hours, taking three more x-rays to check on the lungs and finding them normal each time, doing everything I knew to help her. The little girl just got sicker and sicker and sicker, and finally I called my senior resident at home around three in the morning. He rushed in.

An hour later, the little girl's heart stopped.

I remember the resident hurriedly trying to put in an arterial line, cutting down on her wrist and her ankle, unable to find an artery. And all the while, I kept thinking about what I had done wrong, what I had overlooked, why I hadn't called my senior resident earlier. Unlike a medical residency, in a surgical residency the lines of authority are clear. The medical students reported to the intern, the intern to the resident, the resident to the senior resident, and the senior resident to the staff surgeon. All you had to do was work hard and be a good, honest reporter, obtain the facts and give them accurately to your superior; the system worked well that way. I knew that. Why hadn't I done it sooner?

There was nothing we could do for the child. A young girl

was dead, and she had died on my service, under my care, while I was in charge. I felt as if I had killed her.

I wanted to quit. The more I thought about her, the more guilty I felt. I did not know then that the guilt would never leave me, that years later I would look at my own children and see the face of that little girl. That I would picture her in my dreams at night to this day. All I knew then was that I felt useless, burned out. Did I really want this to be my life?

I had only had six days of vacation that first year. Not much, considering that we had to work every day and all night every other night. I took my vacation around Christmas and went home to Nashville. Dad and I talked about the experience with the little girl, and he told me tales of his own and kept at me, gently and lovingly, to go back, stick it out, and make up for what I thought I had done by becoming the best surgeon possible.

I shared the experience with my brother Bobby, seven years my senior and an experienced cardiac surgeon, who reinforced what Dad had said, wisely reminding me that death, that nature's course, was not always within our control. But I still remember her gentle face and my sense of helplessness and guilt. As always, I listened to both Dad and Bobby. I went on with my plans for school and with Katie. Despite the pressures, despite our problems, later that week Katie and I announced our upcoming wedding in the Nashville papers. The date was set for June.

Back in Boston, when I asked for an additional week off to get married, I was told there would be no other interns available to cover the service in my absence. It was felt to be inappropriate to get married during the first year of a surgical residency. Residency was not designed with the happy home life of newlyweds in mind. It was suggested I wait at least a year. I must have thought this attitude ridiculous even then, but I never admitted it. I had no choice, I thought, but to nod, smile, and go out and work around the system. It would be hard, but I was a surgeon in training and I had penance to do. It never occurred to me to stand up and say what I thought.

Katie and I went ahead with our plans, and I said I would find the time somehow to make it to the wedding, although a honeymoon was out. In April I flew down for twenty-four hours for a wedding party. Four hours down, four back, eight hours more or less asleep, eight hours socializing. Absurd. Crazy. No way to spend your life. No way to get married. Already, I had my doubts, but it took a late-night walk along the Charles River for me to face up to them.

For, finally, it was not the pressures of medical school, nor Katie's career, nor an occasional relationship with other women, nor the stress and guilt of my residency that led me to admit I wanted out of the future Katie and I had planned together for more than a decade. It was Karyn.

I fell in love with her. That's all there was to it. She was all I wanted in life.

I had met Karyn only a few weeks before the planned wedding. But I felt as if I'd known her all my life. I couldn't get the first day out of my mind. I remembered how it started, at the hospital. She came to the emergency room with a sprained wrist. Then the telephone call a few days later. Saying I would come that evening to see her. The west-Texas lilt in her voice when she told me to come ahead. The terrible part of Boston she lived in. Columbus Avenue. A one-bedroom walk-up on the second floor. Her white dress. Her sunburnt face. Her big, wide eyes. How she laughed at me, chided me for my cheapness when I first suggested that we walk to Charlestown, then that we hitchhike. Warren Tavern. The dinner. The conversation. The chemistry. The late evening walk along the Charles River.

And I remembered the rest of the night, too.

I flew down to Nashville two days before the wedding. I had just finished a forty-eight-hour shift at Mass. General. I was still dressed in my white hospital pants, tired, stretched to the limit, blunted emotionally, staring blankly into the long, dark tunnel of the wrong future. It would be years before I could fully assesss the trauma medical school was doing to my soul, but it would be even longer before I could face the memory of what I did that day, like fingering a long, hard, surgical scar and wondering how much had been cut out inside. I had come home to call off the marriage.

Mother picked me up at the airport and took me to see Dad, and I remember how suprisingly well they took the news, news that must have been awful for them, disconcerting and upsetting. Still, they gave me their support, pretended that they were in some way relieved, though there had never been even the slightest hint that they thought anything was amiss. It must have been hard, because even to my ears the excuses that I used, excuses that I would repeat, over and over, sounded hollow. Everyone listened carefully to what I said, all the lame explanations I had that were and were not the truth, and they nodded and dealt with it and I went on my way.

And I remember the house Katie lived in. The gloom that had settled over it as I mouthed words I only half-believed. Long table after table covered with white cloths. Gifts lined up. Plates. Silverware. A large silver bowl. I sat with Katie in the living room on the long sofa, its soft pattern of flowers familiar to me from a thousand other nights we'd spent sharing our feelings. I explained that nothing was right with my life. With me. With me and her. I cried. And she cried, and I stayed an hour, and I flew back to Boston the next morning.

I must have been numb, but it was a condition that by then seemed natural. I was still in those hospital whites. I headed straight to the hospital from the airport. My next shift was starting. I kept thinking about Katie's chocolate brown eyes. I had not mentioned Karyn. I did not miss a minute of work at Mass. General.

5

Nothing much changed at Mass. General during the second, third, and fourth years, except that the training got even more rigorous and demanding. I rotated through the various surgical specialties. I took on more patients. I learned to live with more stress. I discovered I was clearly drawn to the most demanding and the most stressful of the services, cardiac surgery.

My mentor and teacher on that service was a big, silver-haired man who was a charismatic and supremely confident surgeon. Socially he was the most gentlemanly and polite of men, with a delightful wife and well-mannered children. In the OR he could be severely demanding.

For my part, I did my work and lost myself in my love of Karyn. We were married while I was at Mass. General and moved into a small townhouse on Beacon Hill. Whenever we could get away, we would fly to Nantucket just to be alone together. When we couldn't do that, I'd take my small 1954 vintage airplane and fly around Boston for a few hours of blessed freedom.

When I got the opportunity to go to England to study thoracic surgery for six months, Karyn and I planned to fly across the Atlantic together in our old twin-engine plane and have the adventure of our life. Instead, we discovered she was pregnant with Harrison, and when the time came we simply couldn't risk it.

If I had to do it all again, I would have borrowed money for the time we spent in England, lived it up a bit more, spent more time out of the hospital, traveled more, and given Karyn the real benefits that a different country and a different culture affords. As it was, we had a wonderful time anyway, and I enjoyed especially the British no-frills approach to surgery, fenced round as they were by socialized medicine.

When I was in Britain, I would see patients on the second day post-op walking around outside the hospital, fully dressed in their street clothes and carrying their chest-tube bottles with them. Back home in the United States, they'd be in their hospital gowns and confined to their beds for at least a week to ten days. While at Mass. General we would take a sputum specimen and send it off to the lab for extensive analysis and culture, the English would just have patients spit into cups every hour or so and see if the amount was increasing or decreasing over time. In the United States, we might administer a bronchodilator called Alupent through an expensive little mask called a nebulizer to loosen up a patient's lung secretions and prevent spasms in his airways. Over there, the patient would inhale vapor through an old red hose running into a half-inch of liquid eucalyptus in a porcelain bottle made a hundred years ago.

There were many such differences, and I came back more aware than ever how high-tech the U.S. approach to medicine had become. I couldn't say that one was better than the other, but my six months in England reminded me once again why I had wanted to become a doctor in the first place. I would think about my father, and his practice, and then about Mass. General and my training. I realized that I had cut myself in half—I was a high-tech surgeon who wanted to have a family doctor's practice.

And then Norman Shumway and the Stanford group showed me how to put the two back together again.

I leaned back in Dad's easy chair and watched the outside lights play along the floor of the den.

"Something the matter, Son?" Dad said.

"Sorry," I said. "Just drifting. Tired I guess. I was just thinking about how medicine has changed."

"You're right about that. You know what the biggest diseases were when I first started treating patients? Typhoid fever, tuberculosis, syphilis. When's the last time you heard of anybody being treated for those? I mean as primary diseases, not a secondary infection from something like AIDS. Now, it's what? Heart disease, cancer, and even those. . . . 'Bout the only thing that hasn't changed in forty years is diabetes."

"I was thinking more about how a doctor spends his time," I said.

"I know one doctor who should spend more time with his family," he smiled.

I laughed. "You're right. It's late. I should be getting home."

"What's troubling you, Billy?"

"I don't know," I said. "My patients, I guess." I saw the light go on in his eyes. "I mean, I have to guard against getting too close, getting too wrapped up in them. After they're transplanted, they depend so much on us anyway. I've got to think about their social life, their habits, their relationships, all that. I mean I've got a young attorney, forty-five years old, six weeks out and he's doing fine. Good-looking guy, well-off, three children and a wife, called the other day and invited me downtown to watch him try his first case since he became ill."

"So what's the problem?"

"He broke up with his wife. Started dating a married woman. They go out all the time. Stay up late. Go to parties, listen to music, drink. He says no, but I think he's smoking again. I think he's missed his medicine a few times. How do I say to him that this woman—she's fine and all that, I know you love her—but your relationship with her is going to kill you?

"It's worse for Jan, my nurse. She's the real buffer between me and the patients, and she gets really involved with them. She is their friend, their confidante, their doctor, their priest. Being so close to them makes it very difficult for her when they have a setback. It will wear her down. I saw it happen to a transplant nurse at Stanford."

"You talk to her?" he asked.

"Not yet. Not really. But that's not the worst of it. You mentioned diabetes. I've got this guy coming in next week, referred to me by a doctor in East Tennessee I've never met and by some rock star. Cardiomyopathy, a very, very sick man. Medically, he's a good candidate, which is why I'm seeing him. He needs a transplant, and quick.

"But he's got severe diabetes, with peripheral vascular disease. And there are potential problems with compliance, I think. He was on the list at Pittsburgh, then backed out when they found a heart for him because he didn't feel so bad then. And he hasn't given up smoking, in spite of being told that he must do so. They tested him for drugs at Pittsburgh and found traces of cocaine. He's a road manager for this rock star, so drugs are available to him. I don't know. I might not list him."

"He's not the first one," Dad said.

"But the others all had severe medical problems. This has got more to do with issues of lifestyle and compliance. He needs a transplant from the medical standpoint. Who am I to be making decisions like this?"

Dad took a deep breath. He looked out the window. Then came the whisper. "You're the man who was trained to make decisions like this. When I was your age, this fellow would have died, pure and simple. Friends of mine have died of the same thing, people I'd known for years, because we couldn't save them. There was nothing we could do. Now we have the know-how to save some of them. Some of them—not all of them. Well, I raised you to make that decision. I raised you, and this society trained you specifically for that purpose, and you spent years learning how to make it.

"But you know that. What bothers you is that this fellow isn't like you. I don't mean he's poor, anything like that. I mean, he doesn't share your values."

"You're right," I said. "I think I might not like him, and that makes it harder. But there are just too few hearts around to give one to somebody who won't take care of it."

"You're who you are, he's who he is. Maybe you're wrong. Maybe he wasn't ready before, and he is now. Who knows? But I do know you, and I know you would never make such a decision frivolously. And I've never known you to make a bad decision in thirty-odd years."

I looked at him, and he met my eyes.

"What about the monkey?" I asked.

"The monkey?"

140

"Don't you remember the monkey? I wanted a monkey so bad, and you wouldn't let me have it. I wanted one for years. Years. We stopped at that place in Florida on one of our family trips, remember, and I cried for a monkey. And you said, 'No.' "

"Didn't Tommy take you down there sometime years later?"

"That's right, Dad, But it was too late, then. I was too old. We went down to Fort Lauderdale. Flew down. And when we got there, he said, 'You still want a monkey?' And I had wanted one for so long, I automatically said yes, so he took me to some kind of side-of-the-road animal farm. But by then I was too old. It's as if it were yesterday. I remember a hundred or so monkeys, climbing all over each other in crowded, loud cages doing disgusting things, covered with their own excrement. I'd outgrown the desire. I said, 'Let's forget it,' and Tommy laughed himself blue in the face."

My father was smiling broadly as he stood up to walk me to the door.

"My point, exactly," he said. "You didn't make the decision until the time was right."

"For you," I said.

"To make the right decision," he said.

We stood at the door for a minute, looking out into the Nashville night, and he put his hand on my shoulder.

"It's the only thing I ever wanted that I didn't get," I said, and we both burst out laughing.

Laughing, I got into my old BMW, started up, and drove away. Laughing, I did not remember feeling good for having made the right choice. I remembered instead the ache. The hollow feeling in my bones. The way a picture of a monkey or the sound of the word actually hurt somehow.

I had not liked that feeling, that longing for something I couldn't have, and driving home from my father's that night I realized why. At the time, I had never had such a feeling before. I couldn't remember when the monkey business had first come up. I must have been nine, maybe ten. Nine or ten, I thought, shaking my head, was the first time in my life I felt *normal*.

Part Four

A DAY IN THE LIVES

1

The year I operated on Jim Hayes was a busy one, a building year. By the anniversary of his operation, we had transplanted some thirty hearts. At one point during that time we had four transplant patients recovering in the intensive-care unit at the same time. There was a lot of activity for a new program. We did three more heart-lung transplants, more than anyone else in the Southeast. All of our patients made it through the operation and almost all of them went back to living active, normal, and productive lives.

But Jean Lefkowitz did not make it. She died not long after my late-night conversation with Dad. As I feared, her death hit the team pretty hard.

In some ways, I was luckier than most of the others. I had been through the deaths of beloved patients at Stanford. And surgeons, as professionals, learn early how to deal with such losses. Either they learn or they get out. One would think medical school would give surgeons handy psychological tools with which to face the inevitable defeats. But there were no such courses. A surgeon learns on his feet, as an apprentice, observing and assimilating the behavior of those around him.

The surgeon's job blunted his sentiments. Even routine surgery, finely tuned as it was, frequently required him to make quick decisions with limited information under dire circumstances. He had to make them without hesitation or fear of mistake, knowing full well that the wrong move, the wrong decision, could mean instant death. A surgeon had to live with that decision, whatever the outcome, and sometimes it was not easy. While surgeons generally were risk-takers, they still needed a certain distance between themselves and their patients in order to perform in an impassioned, deliberate, and focused manner. The rigid hierarchy around the operating table, the very necessary servile attention to the surgeon's every command and move, the careful dehumanization of the surgical field—all the rituals of the operating theater were aimed in part at creating and maintaining that distance, at reinforcing the surgeon's sense of control and confidence, at allowing him to walk away when a patient died and operate another day.

The nature of surgery itself afforded the physician the opportunity to view patients to some degree as a series of cases, technical events in the course of his work. Even postoperative care could remain more or less abstract, a series of charts and computerized reports calling for this or that adjustment. It may have seemed inhumane, but it did provide surgeons a certain functional insularity.

I could always come out of the operating room feeling I had done my professional best. For some surgeons, of course, it ended there. They indulged in the aura of infallibility created by the system and arrogantly avoided dealing with patients to any significant degree beyond the operation. As my father's son, trained in the tradition of Norman Shumway and Ed Stinson, I knew there was a vast distance between being paralyzed by guilt and feeling like the fastest draw in the West.

Transplant surgery discouraged gunslingers. The transplant surgeon was not finished when he tied the last stitch. In fact, that was just the beginning. He was never done with his patients. When a nontransplant surgical patient left the hospital after an operation, he maybe saw his surgeon for a single postdischarge visit and that was it. When a transplant patient did well, he developed a long-term relationship with his surgeon. The lifelong commitment to a patient's postoperative care was one of the things that attracted me to transplantation, but it also meant I had to find new ways to keep the distance necessary for me to continue to function when I did lose one of my chimeras.

At Stanford, I had learned to use the Great Wall for that purpose. What had once seemed something of a personal handicap became a professional advantage.

On the one hand, I accepted the fact that intimacy would never come easily for me, that I might never find outside of Karyn and my family even one close friend like the close friends others seemed to have—someone I trusted and cherished beyond the mutual respect that comes from sharing a profession or the easy camaraderie of a common background.

On the other hand, I knew I could treat others, especially patients, with more than courtesy, with a certain warmth and compassion, even tenderness, because the wall was always there when I needed it. Behind it lay my real world, Karyn and the kids—a world emotionally free of the job. Despite the long hours and the exhausting nature of my work, I could quickly retreat to my inner world if the sudden deaths or the inexorable sufferings proved too much for me. For Karyn and the kids, for my family, I knew I could even turn my back on my profession.

Unlike surgeons, nurses did not have the institutionally supported luxury of avoiding postoperative care, of setting themselves beyond human contact with recovering mortals. Not that nurses weren't professionals in the full sense of the word. They were also trained to view the patient as a medical case, to pay close attention to charts, to watch for clinical signs of improvement or danger. But in their role as minute-to-minute caretakers, nurses spent much more time with patients than even the most dedicated surgeons. If they didn't actually make the life-or-death decisions about patient treatment that the surgeons made, nurses nevertheless spent many hours implementing those decisions. And they called the shots in a thousand and one smaller ways concerning a patient's daily comfort and care.

But nurses were also trained to treat patients as human beings. The better they were at their jobs, the more a patient became an individual, a real person with his own special needs and wants, someone with a history greater than the terse summaries written in the medical record, with a family, with hopes and dreams, with foibles and quirks, with feelings and emotions, with a voice and face and expressions and manners they recognized and remembered afterward. When a patient died, nurses couldn't turn to the surgical litany, "cut well, tie well, get well; after that it's out of my hands," to help them face that death. They had to do it on their own.

The average intensive-care nurse lasted less than four years on the job. We did not yet have comparable statistics on heart-transplant nurses, but my guess was their record would be even worse. Nurses in transplant programs had even more direct responsibility for their patients than nurses in other units. Their patients stayed longer, required more detailed attention, took more medicines, needed more tests, suffered a wider variety of medical problems, had more psychological adjustments, and got sicker more suddenly and for more obscure reasons than most other patients.

Transplant recipients not only had to learn which of the many medicines to take and when, they also had to learn all about how their new heart worked. Since those hearts did not have nerves and pain fibers running to the brain, the recipients would not feel pain, even when the heart was ischemic, hungry for blood and oxygen. Such transplanted hearts, though as strong and powerful as nontransplanted hearts, did not respond quite as quickly when patients started to exercise. In the ICU, transplant patients learned for the first time how to adapt to such idiosyncrasies, to warm up their hearts before trying to walk up stairs, to be on the lookout for trouble by being aware of symptoms more subtle than chest pain.

Transplant nurses not only tended their patients but taught them.

Transplant nurses saw things other nurses might not normally see: a man euphoric in the morning, bawling like a baby at night; a woman strong and healthy and ready to go home one day, near death and back on the respirator the next; minor irritations—cold sores, skin rashes, raw spots—spreading across a patient's body like some deadly, unknown disease. They learned not to trust their former experience, to ignore appearances; they had to be on their guard constantly, to question everything, to expect surprise. The temptation was to make each transplant patient a personal cause; the danger in doing so, emotional burn-out.

I knew what could happen to transplant nurses, and I knew how strongly our folks had felt about Jean Lefkowitz. The week she died I made a special effort to keep an eye on Holley Cully, who worked with transplants on the Seven North step-down unit and who had been Jean's primary-care nurse.

Holley was an open, friendly young woman who had taken to transplant care like a duck to water. She had a good feel for the work, and I kept her informed and sought her opinion when I made rounds. She had a young son at home whom she talked about often, a sense of humor, and a hard-headed approach to life that I found refreshing. She talked openly about Jean's death, but she seemed more angry than depressed. Each time I oh-so-deli-cately questioned her about it, she appeared to be on the verge of saying something but then drawing back.

Finally, I said, "OK, Holley. What is it?"

"What?"

"About Jean. What is it you want to say?"

"It's nothing, really," she said. I waited her out. "I don't know if I should." I stepped away from the station, where the usual crowd of residents, interns, nurses, and receptionists were sitting around, watching electronic blips on television screens, looking over charts, and gossiping. Holley followed me.

"It just makes me so angry," she said.

"What makes you angry?"

"I guess you wouldn't know. How could you? You don't hear what they're saying."

"Who? What who's saying?"

"The nurses on the other floors. Doctors. People here in the hospital."

"No," I said. "I haven't heard what they're saying, but I can guess."

In fact, I did know. In the closed world of a hospital, gossip circulated like recycled air through every ward and floor. You didn't have to hear it exactly, you more or less breathed it in.

"They" were saying that we shouldn't do heart-lungs; that the operations were too experimental; that that was the reason Jean had died. And "they" were saying that the transplant program was doomed to fail; that it was too expensive; that it cost the hospital too much; that other areas and other patients were suffering because of it. "They" were saying that our success rate really wasn't all that good; that the whole thing was mainly for show; and that the only reason I was here at all was because my Dad ran HCA, my brother was a prominent surgeon, and my family had influence in town.

"They" were saying the very things I had always dreaded hearing, the things I had spent half my life trying to prove weren't true, the things that caused me to leave Nashville years before.

"They just don't know," Holley said, as if she had read my mind. Instead, I knew, she was simply speaking her own. "They pick up on someone like Jean, but they never look at a James Bunning, a Jimmy Moore, a Charles Mullins, a Mark Johnson, or any of the others that are doing well. They don't know anything about organ donation or transplantation or anything, about how you travel around to educate people and all that. They just see you on TV and get mad."

"It takes time," I laughed. "Even here. You just stick with me and look after these patients, and in a year—two at the most—you will single-handedly have made this place as good as any transplant center in the world."

"Give me a break," she said and slapped my shoulder. As I turned to go, she stopped me. "Dr. Frist, I am incredibly depressed about Jean, and I know what you are trying to do. I'm not stupid. And don't you worry, I'm going to be fine. That doesn't mean you can stop coming around here, asking me what I think, and telling me how great my ideas are, though."

We both laughed, and I left much relieved.

I was also worried about Jan Muirhead, and she was much more difficult for me to approach than Holley.

Jan had been around a lot longer than I had. She was from Memphis, the daughter of a prominent pathologist, and she had come out of the University of Kentucky nursing school to take a job in Vanderbilt's surgical intensive-care unit. From there, she went to work for Harvey Bender, chief of the Department of Cardiac and Thoracic Surgery, before she left for Seattle to earn a master's at the University of Washington.

In the meanwhile, Harvey had hired Walter Merrill, who in time would become my surgical associate. The two of them were planning a heart-transplant program just about the time Jan finished up out West. They persuaded her to come back to Nashville, head the nursing end of the program, and serve as a coordinator for the patients. She had accepted the job in January, then tried to attend one of the first instructional transplant conferences at Stanford in February. But it was too late for her to register. She knew next to nothing about the field when she began her new job at Vanderbilt in March.

The program already had one patient on its waiting list. During Jan's first week on the job nervous nurses called her and anxiously asked when they were going to be trained. She threw herself—in typical Muirhead fashion—headlong into the task, constantly studying, skipping sleep altogether, totally dedicating herself to learning all she could about transplantation as quickly as possible. She managed to plan the in-services program and to write the nursing protocols before a donor was found. She did a good job, despite the limited time she had.

I met her later that year at another Stanford conference. I had already accepted the position at Vanderbilt, but I had not yet left California. I realized immediately that she was quite a find. Vanderbilt had conducted five heart transplants at that point, but two of the patients had died, and she made no bones about the program's shortcomings and inexperience. She didn't flatter me, but she made it clear she was glad Vanderbilt had hired me. She wanted to learn to do things right, she said, to follow the Stanford model, which of course pleased me. She was obviously willing to invest her life in the program.

No one on staff was more excited than Jan a year later when we did our first heart-lung transplant operation on Jean Lefkowitz. Like Walter, Harvey, and me, she felt she had a lot at stake in the program and that the operation would put us on the map. But she had even more riding on the operation than we did, because she got to know Jean better.

Partly, it was in the nature of her job. It was Jan who met with patients after I interviewed them to walk them step by step through the whole procedure. She helped them figure out their finances, the arrangements they should make for home care, whether they were better off working or going on disability. She got them their beepers, answered their questions, and booked local rooms when they needed them. She sat with patients before surgery and with their families during the operation. She met with patients during their postoperative stay in the hospital, scheduling their trips to physical therapy and coordinating their care with our nutritionist, our psychiatrist, our social worker. She set up their trips to the clinic after they had left the hospital and met with them each time, checking their progress, their physical condition, and their compliance with the therapy. She became familiar with almost every aspect of their personal lives, including the intimate details.

But part of it, too, was Jan's personality. She was a woman who defined her existence almost exclusively by her work. Her time was dedicated entirely to the lives of others. She had almost no private life and few relationships outside the job; she believed she could not do her work well otherwise. She spent every moment she could at the hospital, and when she took time off, she worried constantly about the patients, afraid she had missed some small something-or-other in their lab work that might cost them their lives, sure that in her absence they had called in dire trouble and that no one had understood the seriousness of the situation.

For all those reasons—Jan's dedication to the program, the nature of her job, and her perfectionism—someone like Jean Lefkowitz easily became dependent on her, sometimes obsessively so. Severely depressed by the breakup of her marriage after her operation, Jean called Jan virtually every day of her life until she returned to Vanderbilt. And then Jean's luck ran out. Jan felt the blow as both a private loss and a professional failure.

For two weeks I watched her struggle with Jean's death, distracted, out of sorts, red-eyed, and I did not really know what to say to her. Because I myself needed something more than my work, because I so valued my marriage and my family, I tended to think that Jan's work was substituting for a meaningful private life and that it was unhealthy, and in the long run detrimental, for her to get so close to the recipients. But even if I was right, that's not what she needed to hear just now.

On the other hand, I was afraid we would lose Jan, if not now, then one day too soon; I had to do something. I had decided to talk to her on Tuesday next, after the clinic, when we had finished seeing our other transplant patients. I would tell her how Jean's death got to me, too, how it hit all of us, maybe even bring up the Great Wall in some fashion or other, help her build at least a chain-link fence.

But before I said anything, she surprised me. I walked into my office after lunch on Tuesday to go over the file on Jimmy Moore with her. He was a patient under my care who had been transplanted at Vanderbilt before I arrived and who was in the clinic that day.

And Jan said, "Jimmy's got big plans. He wants to take Al Moore and some of the others and bicycle clean across Tennessee during Organ Donor Awareness Week this year."

"Like Jim Hayes."

"Un-huh. Like Jim Hayes."

"I don't know," I said. Then I saw the gleam in her eye, the smile hidden behind her expression. "You think I should let him."

"I think he might do it anyway if you don't," she said, and her smile broke out into the open.

"What? What is it?"

"I want to go with them," she said.

153

2

Jimmy Moore had just completed a triathlon, and he was depressed. It was the same old thing.

He hated the way people at work and at home treated him as if he were some kind of invalid, like a puny, helpless little child no matter what feat of physical strength and endurance he pulled off. He was the same man he was before he received a transplant over a year ago, the same rugged sport he was before he got sick, when he had literally climbed mountains for relaxation from his construction job and his volunteer work on the rescue squad in his South Carolina hometown.

He could look in the mirror and see himself as he was, as he had always been, his long, reddish hair brushed back from a high forehead, his red beard outlining a strong, square jaw, his moustache softening the severity of his aquiline nose—a handsome, muscular, virile man in his late twenties. He could do anything they could do and do it better than most of them. Why didn't they see that?

They treated him like he was in some kind of glass cage. It had started the minute he got home from his stay in Nashville, after a month spent in the hospital, a month in that claustrophobic halfway house where he had to live in one small room and a kitchen. He hadn't seen much of his young children, who stayed at home with Robin, their mother, and he hadn't been able to go out at all at first, except to walk two blocks over to the hospital each day for his physical therapy with Jay Groves.

Jimmy smiled. He liked Jay Groves, a fit little guy with longish wiry hair who was in charge of Vanderbilt Hospital's rehab program and who reminded him of that exercise nut—Richard Simmons, right?—on television. And he liked the time he spent

154

downstairs in the rehab center with the other heart patients and transplants, working through his routine, running in place, bicycling. It had kept him from going crazy, locked in that room with nothing to do but read the newspaper or watch TV.

Holley Cully had helped a lot, both before and after the operation. She and Jimmy and Robin had become great friends, and Holley would drop by and go out to dinner with them when Robin got away from the kids and work and came up to stay for a few days. The dinners weren't so hot because they had to go at odd hours and sit off by themselves and he had to wear that stupid blue mask and people stared, but it was nice to get out anyway. And sometimes Holley would just come over and sit and talk, and then he remembered what it was like to feel normal.

He looked forward to going home and feeling that way all the time, but it didn't happen like that. There were all the medicines to take, of course, and you had to constantly check your temperature, and watch your diet, and all that kind of thing, but it was no worse really than being like somebody from California who followed all the latest health fads. In fact, it just meant he was in better shape health-wise than he'd been before all this happened.

And there were the little surprises. He couldn't mow the lawn. For some reason, he was unable to push the lawn mower like he used to. Already he could lift just about anything he wanted, and he was beginning to work out with weights, something he had never done before, but when it came to cutting the grass. . . .

If he'd been Robin, he would have been suspicious, figuring that he was using the operation as an excuse to get out of doing a chore he disliked. But his wife was so sure he was still a sick weakling that she just accepted it, despite everything else he could do.

Things like that only reminded him of when he was a kid and had asthma and couldn't run. He had never been able to run, really, but he had done everything else, swum a lot, played basketball, climbed mountains—how was it any different now? So he bought himself one of those tractor mowers and went out on

155

Saturdays and rode around all morning mowing the lawn. And then Robin had called his brothers, who had rushed down to his house and jumped all over him.

Sure, he had days, especially at first, when he felt rundown and beat, but then he also had days when he felt great, as if he could do anything, as if the heart inside his chest was the one he had been born with and it had never gone bad. But it didn't matter. People still wouldn't smoke around him. If he bumped into them out walking, they'd say, "Hey, you look really great, but don't you overdo it now."

Everybody in his town knew who he was and felt as if they had some kind of stake in his life. He'd see them coming out of the bank, and they'd look at his car, and say, "How come you're out driving? Why are you by yourself? Where's Robin? Why isn't she with you?" Some of them tried to be more subtle. "My, it's hot out here today, don't you think?" But the message was clear.

He hadn't expected to go back to work right away, of course, but he didn't see why he couldn't continue with his volunteer activities at the rescue squad. Oh, they let him come around, but they wouldn't let him do anything. They'd been kinder back when he got sick. Then, at least, they let him be dispatcher for a while. He had been secretary-treasurer as well, and they kept that open for him when he went for his stay at Vanderbilt. Some other guy stepped in for a while, but when he got home they said, "Here, this is all your responsibility."

He thought at first that meant he was really back on the squad, and the first time his beeper went off he rushed from his house down to the wreck. Normally, he would have gone to headquarters, but the accident was closer to his house than the squad garage, so he showed up at the scene. What a mistake. They all just looked at him, then took him aside and said, "You're going to hurt yourself. We don't want you to get hurt." Like it was going to kill him to stand there and put a bandage on somebody.

And then his friend who ran the squad took him out for a drink. "Jimmy," he said. "I've got to be honest with you. We don't want you out on call, driving a truck, or anything like that. I mean, with all that medication you're on, if something did happen. You're out there traveling seventy, eighty miles per hour in an emergency truck, sirens going and all, and somebody hits you. They use that in a court of law against you. You were driving, you're on medication, it's your fault."

What the hell, they acted like he was diabetic or something, as if he was going to go into some kind of shock from the steroids. But it was no use, he thought. They just didn't understand. He moped around the house for a while after that, depressed, thinking about all he had been through.

He remembered how suddenly he had gotten sick. Just one day going to the doctor, and the doctor said he had the flu. Go home. Slow down. Rest. Drink plenty of liquids. What a hoot. Two days later, he went back to the doctor and said he wasn't getting any better, and again they said it was flu. We've seen a lot of this kind of thing. It's going around. Yeah. Right. Then he was throwing up and totally fatigued, and the old hometown doc finally decided to do a complete checkup, blood tests, x-rays, the works.

They showed him his heart on the x-ray, and it scared him silly. It was huge. He couldn't remember the first time someone mentioned the word "transplant," but he certainly remembered going up to Vanderbilt for a second opinion. And the tests. The IVs were bad enough, but the needles. They stuck needles in his feet. He was a strong person, but the needles in his feet were more than he could take. When Vanderbilt agreed that he needed a transplant, they said he had his choice of where to get it, but there was never any choice, really. Anywhere else, he'd have to go through those tests again, and he wasn't about to do that.

And then, oh God, the wait. At first they wouldn't even put him on the list because he was so sick, and Robin was really scared, crying all the time and praying. He had a pulmonary embolus, a clot in his lungs, so they put him in the local hospital and postponed everything for a few weeks while they dissolved the clot. Then, when he was well enough to travel, they took him up to Vanderbilt; he was still too sick to go on the list for another week or so.

At first he thought it was going to be fine. Holley picked him up at the airport, and sick as he was, they decided to go to dinner, one last big meal before D-day. He took a nitroglycerine tablet to get through it, and then another one during dinner, and another when he arrived at the Vanderbilt admitting office. In his room, he took a fourth. He was starting to feel a lot better, thinking maybe he wouldn't have to have an operation after all.

And he did get better, and they put him on the list, and he thought, Oh, boy, what for? But the wait had started. It lasted five weeks, and he grew worse each day, his heart growing bigger and flabbier by the minute. *Five weeks.* He lay there, or sat there, or paced there in the hospital room, sick as a dog, weak as a kitten, thinking he wasn't going to make it, that he would never go rock-climbing again, or hiking, or riding his motorcycle, never make love to Robin, never see the kids graduate or get married or have kids of their own.

Four weeks in, they came and said, "We think we have a heart. Call your wife." And Robin drove up, while he paced around his room for twelve hours, psyching himself up, thinking, This is it, this is it. And then they came in and said, "No go." It disgusted him, it disappointed him, it scared the hell out of him. He found out from Holley that they had tried out two hearts that day; one didn't match and the other belonged to a guy who had hepatitis. He was sure his luck had run out. If he hadn't had Robin and the two kids, if they weren't counting on him, if they hadn't been so brave, he'd have found some way to kill himself rather than lie there and suffer any longer.

Robin came up the next week, and the two of them went out for dinner, both of them thinking it was their last supper, neither of them much wanting to talk about it. They had three hours. Alone. All to themselves. They had just walked out the door when the resident came flying down the stairs looking for them. As he raced outside, they climbed into their Trans Am and pulled out of the parking space. He was running across the street toward the parking lot when they paid their ticket and pulled off, leaving him behind in their rearview mirror, his white coattails flapping, his waving hands held high.

158

Jimmy remembered the bedlam he walked into three hours later. Jan, Holley, the residents, all of them were frantic. They had his heart. They pushed him upstairs. They had to check him out, they said. Run tests. Make sure he was up to par. Obtain a chest x-ray, run an ECG, do some blood tests. They flung him down in a wheelchair, said, "Let's go," and took off. Some guy came at the last minute, stuck a sheet of paper in front of him, and said, "Here. You need to sign this consent form."

Jimmy's nerves were shot. "OK," he said. "Fine. I'll sign it."

"No, no. You need to read it first."

"I don't have to read it, God damn it," Jimmy said. "I've already read it. I read it weeks ago. I understand it. It says I might die and it ain't your fault. OK. OK."

Jimmy looked at Jan. "Get this guy out of here," he said. "Get him out! Tell him to forget it! Just forget it, for Christ's sake. I'm not gonna do it. It's going too fast. I'm not gonna do it."

Jimmy realized, of course, how stupid all that was. If Dr. Rodeheffer, who was the transplant cardiologist at that point, had not come in and calmed him down and gotten him to sign the paper and go ahead as planned, he knew he'd most likely die soon. And as it was, he almost didn't make it anyway. He had that seizure in intensive care, that grand mal thing.

Was that ever frustrating. He'd been laughing and joking around with the nurse, and there she was standing outside the room, looking in and drinking her Coke, because they were short-handed and she had stepped out for a quick break, took her mask off, looking at him, smiling, and he was waving his hand, and she was waving back at him, and his leg was jumping up and down, shaking, and it wouldn't stop, and he was waving at her, and she was laughing.

He woke up in a coffin. Only lights were flashing, and he couldn't move, and he suddenly realized he was alive, but he didn't know where he was or what was happening. And then there were people all around him, saying, "Calm down, Mr. Moore, calm down," and he said, "What are you talking about?" and someone said, "You just had a transplant." He thought they

159

were trying to kill him. Cut him up for spare parts. That he was in the middle of a Frankenstein movie. And he tried to get up, striking out with his fists, his feet, anything to keep them from killing him. "You're wife's out there," they said. "I'm not married!" he screamed. Later, he found out they'd been trying to do a CT scan of his brain.

And he had lived through it all, and gotten better, and come home feeling good and normal. But no one believed it.

Sometime during that first month back home, Jimmy Moore realized he was driving himself deeper and deeper into a real fugue of a depression by just sitting around thinking about everything that had happened to him. He decided to fight back. He got together with his closest buddies and went mountain climbing. He took along his video equipment and made a home movie and started showing it to everybody who would watch, including his doctors.

They hit the ceiling. And when they "jumped on him," as Jimmy would say, he jumped right back. He told them that they were always talking about "quality of life" and a "functional lifestyle," and he was taking them at their word. They, of all people, should not treat him like a freak. And he announced he was going to enter a triathlon. And he started training for it in the middle of Main Street in his hometown. He did it deliberately so that everyone could see him and know what he was doing.

That was about the time that he became my patient, four months into his new life. I recognized right away that I had a volatile man on my hands, one with a lot of pride and a strong will. He was a fighter who for the first time in his life found himself the member of an oppressed minority, battling to live up to the potential he knew he had but that others, through ignorance, denied him. I was on his side in that battle, and I encouraged him—within limits—to enter the race.

One thing he knew from his days in the hospital was that he should not swim in lakes because the risk of infection was too high. At my urging, he searched long and hard for a triathlon in Tennessee that held its swimming competition in a pool. He couldn't find one, and he showed up at his monthly visit to the clinic very down in the mouth, sure that I would take him out of the running.

"I don't believe I want my patient swimming around in Percy Priest Lake," I said.

He wouldn't look me in the eye. He and Jan exchanged quick glances, then Jimmy got red in the face, biting back his anger, staring off at the opposite wall.

I slapped him on the knee, stood up, and said, "I can't stand that hangdog look you get. All right. Here's what we do. Before the triathlon, before you get anywhere near a body of water of any kind whatsoever outside of an empty pool, we pump you so full of antibiotics that no self-respecting germ will come near you."

That was ten months ago. He had been in two more triathlons since; in the last one he had had other heart-transplant patients running with him, one of them Mark Johnson. The two were quite a pair, one a deer hunter, one a mountain climber, both trying to prove to themselves that they were, in fact, cured of not just heart disease but also of their own doubts. They hadn't feared much of anything until they had found themselves facing certain death; now they were normal again and they wanted to revel in it.

For Mark it was easier. He had a job to go back to, his family's business, and his days were filled with work and his young wife and his own deep, abiding religious faith. For Jimmy Moore, the stakes got higher each time. He had proved his point with the first triathlon. Everybody he knew was stunned and amazed that a heart-transplant patient could do what he was doing. But they couldn't shake off their prejudices.

No one would give him a job. He knew better than to try to look for construction work again; he could imagine the laughter that would have caused among the tough boys laying bricks and hammering nails. But he was perfectly capable of doing almost anything else, and he had always been fascinated by law enforcement.

The police wouldn't have him. They didn't come right out and say they thought he was a cripple, but they failed to hide their

161

surprise that a heart-transplant patient would even think of chasing crooks, or catching speeders, or writing parking tickets for heaven's sake. It was the same line he had gotten from the rescue squad.

Then he checked out other possibilities in sales, in merchandising, even hustling used cars. He was acquainted with most of the people he approached, and he was deeply hurt when they turned him down—especially an old buddy at a local car shop, a guy he'd gone through high school with, grown up with.

"I'd like to help you, Jimmy," the friend said. "But I've got my other employees to think about and my business. If I hired you, my insurance would go sky-high, and I just can't afford it."

"Yeah, sure," Jimmy said.

Recently, finally, he had found something. He was now working as a sort of PR man for the local Chamber of Commerce, recruiting new businesses that came to town into the ranks. But I sensed it was not a very challenging job, not the kind of job Jimmy wanted. It had a limited future, and it smacked of make-work. I was afraid that Jimmy would give it up in disgust.

For he was in a pattern of sorts, demanding too much of himself, always wanting to do more to prove himself, trying to live what he called a normal life. If doing so had just been a matter of physical ability and honest pluck, Jimmy would have excelled, but it's not. Society is not fair—in the way Jimmy wanted it to be—to anyone, really, whether they were a transplant patient or not. But for Jimmy that basic unfairness had gotten tied up with his self-image as a transplant patient.

Lots of people have trouble finding meaningful work, or getting others to see them as they are, or setting goals that work for them, but in Jimmy's case—as in the case of oppressed minorities everywhere—it was clearly complicated by prejudice against him. Part of Jimmy still refused to accept that he was a transplant patient, and it was as destructive as someone blaming himself for the color of his skin. It led to an all but conscious self-loathing. He needed his physical challenges, I knew, to keep him from hating himself. They were his personal march on Selma.

He would try to live a normal life, be rebuffed, and go into training for another triathlon. He'd work hard, push himself to the limit mentally and physically, show up at the event so excited that his legs shook, swim six-tenths of a mile, ride a bike for twenty-five miles, then run-walk-run-walk the six and two-tenths mile run. Afterward, he would come to his next clinic visit so depressed he could hardly talk.

"What is it, Dr. Frist?" he'd say. "I don't even look like a transplant. My cheeks don't puff at all."

And he kept trying until he won. I was incredibly proud of him when I saw the news of his victory on television that night. I called to tell him so. I gathered from what he said that every other member of the transplant team and most of the patients had called too. But I suspected that come the first Tuesday of next month, either he would be further down in the dumps than ever or he would have arrived at some other scheme, more grandiose than a triathlon.

I had no idea which it would be until Jan told me that she wanted to go bike riding halfway across kingdom come with him.

"No," I said. "I don't think it's a good idea."

Jimmy Moore was getting that look on his face.

"But—," he said.

"It's one thing," I said, "to go swimming and riding and jumping and running around at a controlled event, where help is just around the corner. But to go pedaling across a state with nobody around to help and no place to go if you get in trouble—Jimmy, it's not twenty-five miles, with people standing cheering you on; it's five hundred miles, with long stretches of deserted road, and huge hills, and cars zipping past. It's too risky."

"Go ahead, say it," he said. "For a heart transplant."

"For anybody. For me. I wouldn't do it."

I think Jimmy was a bit surprised by his own heat. He must have heard the bitterness in his own voice, because he seemed to take a step back, somehow, even though he was sitting on the

163

edge of the bed in the examining room. He looked to Jan for support, and she steadfastly refused to make eye contact.

"But I won't be alone. Al's going."

"Good, that means two of you can wind up in a ditch mangled by a Mack truck."

"And Jan. She'll take care of us."

"I need Jan right here taking care of my more sensible patients."

"Like Jim Hayes? He bicycled across the entire country, for Pete's sake."

"That's right. And I read his book about the trip, and it sent chills down my spine. If he'd been my patient at Stanford, I wouldn't have let him do it either."

It was miracle Jim Hayes had survived the trip. He and his brother fought driving rain through Kentucky and Missouri, had a serious accident outside Saint Louis, just barely managed to avoid being frozen to death by a snowstorm in the Rockies. It was a rousing, inspiring story, and you couldn't help but admire Jim Hayes for his daring, but it had been a stupid thing to do.

I was not opposed to Jimmy's triathlons. In fact, I had encouraged Mark Johnson and the young attorney I had mentioned to my dad, Al Moore (no relation to Jimmy), to get involved with them. Exercise was good for my patients, the discipline of training for the event good for them, too. And the contests were excellent opportunities to advertise the fact that transplant patients were in no way physically handicapped.

But we could control such events to some extent, arrange with the organizers to allow health professionals to check up on the transplant patients between heats. We strapped heart monitors around their chests, which measured their heart rates as they competed; the monitors beeped loudly through special watches on their wrists if those rates went too high. We had teams standing by to take over in case of emergency. I didn't worry that Jimmy or Mark or Al could not make the trip Jimmy proposed, but I did worry that we did not have the technology to provide a safety net for them over such a long distance.

That's what had struck me about Jim Hayes's description of his trip across country to Stanford—how alone he was, even with his brother by his side. I had winced my way through most of the book, thinking of all the risks he had taken so blithely, awed by the bounty of a merciful Providence for letting him off without so much as a single sniffle. Nobody, but nobody, had Jim Hayes's luck, and I feared God simply would not let another transplant patient get away with something like that.

"Look, Dr. Frist," Jimmy Moore said. "I'm not just doing this for me. Sure, sure, I'm doing it for me. I'm not saying that. But I'm doing it, too, to get attention, you know, for transplants. Just like Jim did with—what was the name of that program?"

" 'That's Incredible!' " Jan said.

" 'That's Incredible!' " Jimmy said. "All the Tennessee stations will pick it up if we let them know. And maybe even the networks if you help us, back us up on this. I've thought this out, I tell you. They'll stay right with us, nothing to worry about."

"No they won't," I said. "Some of them will be there to see you off, then they'll take their little minicams, or whatever they call them, and hop in their vans, and drive to Nashville, sit around having drinks, then film you coming into town, huffing and puffing, all red in the face, and try to get your dying breath on tape after you collapse right in front of them from another grand-mal seizure."

Jimmy and Jan both guffawed. "You sure are a cynical son of a gun," Jimmy said. "Must be the medical training."

"No," I said. "I just read Jim Hayes's book."

"It's not only me," Jimmy said, serious again. "Not just Mark, either. We were all out front there, talking and all, you know, before you came in. There's lots of them who want to go. Al, that attorney guy? He wants to go. And Ron."

"Ron?"

"Yeah. Ron Wynn. You know, the—"

"Ron Wynn wants to go?" I said, incredulous. I looked at Jan, and she shrugged, looking a bit startled herself.

"Bunch of 'em do," Jimmy said. "We could pass out donor

cards everywhere we went. It'd be good for the program." He was smiling big now, like the used-car man he had once wanted to be. "Morale, and all that stuff."

"It will not be good for the program." I said, "when all of you get pneumonia."

"There go the two-year survival statistics," Jan piped up.

Both of us looked at her. Everything was silent for a second. Then we all burst out laughing.

"Look, Dr. Frist," Jimmy said. "Will you do me a favor? Will you not say no right now? Will you just think it over a little? Talk to some of the other ones about it?"

"I'll think about it," I said. I watched as both Jimmy's and Jan's eyes gleamed, glancing back and forth for a moment or two, little twinkles of recognition that said, Ah, we've hooked our sucker now. And I added, "But I'm not making any promises."

On the way down the hall to see our next patient, I leaned down next to Jan's ear and whispered, "This is your fault."

3

I wanted to make sure that the next patient I saw had not been one of those standing out front earlier talking with Jimmy Moore about this latest crazy test of his manhood. I needed to put off thinking about the bike trip for a while. When we walked into the office behind the clinic's reception area, Jan marched over to one of the empty desks where she had the folders for each of the patients arranged in a tidy, overlapping line—probably in alphabetical order, I thought.

"Who do you want to see now?" she asked.

"Well, let's think about that for a minute. Let's see, who's here? Is Hal Buckley in today? Hal Buckley."

Jan handed me Hal's file. "He's due for his first biopsy since he checked out," she said. "We didn't get it this morning, so we rescheduled him for later today, after you've seen him. We got everything else. His creatinine's fine, heart rate normal, blood pressure 120/70, weight about the same—seventy-five kilos."

"How's he doing?" I asked.

"Well," she said and paused, being careful what she said. "He's taking all his medicines, right on schedule, keeping good track of them. Swears he's not gone back to smoking, and I believe him because his wife backs him up. Says he's watching what he eats, exercising regularly. Hasn't any complaints really about side effects. To hear him tell it, everything's going fine."

"But."

"But, there's something going on there. Between him and his wife, or psychologically, I don't know. When you go in to see him, try to figure it out." Jan in her usual way had sensed that something was not quite right.

"He's a tough one to deal with, isn't he?" I said.

"Yes. And I don't really understand it."

"He reminds me a lot of some surgeons I know," I said.

Jan laughed. "That's it. That's it. He wants to—"

"—take control," I said.

"He's read up on transplantation, almost gone overboard in searching out all the details, and he's asking all kinds of questions about the drugs. Like prednisone. Wants to know if we can lower the dosage further because it might be damaging his liver.

"And he's driving himself nuts. He's collected all the survival statistics, knows just what his chances are to survive two years, five years. He's scared out of his wits but won't admit it. I think we're going to have compliance problems with him, especially if he thinks he can start adjusting his own medicines. He's not the kind of guy you'd prefer to transplant under normal circumstances."

Under normal circumstances, I thought, we wouldn't have had to transplant him. He had come to us from another hospital in the area, the victim of a massive heart attack. Every single one of the coronary arteries that wreathed his heart like vines were blocked beyond repair. He did not respond to the conventional therapy for heart attacks, nor to the hottest high-tech treatments. He was going to die, and there wasn't much time. He shot to the top of the transplant list the minute we placed him on it because he was going downhill so fast. By one of those weird throws of the dice we found him a heart that matched the very next day. As far as he was concerned, less than a week before he had been a perfectly healthy forty-three-year-old executive, and now—suddenly—he was a chimera.

But if I had seen him the Saturday night before at the party he had been attending, if I had talked to him for even the briefest time about his job and his life, I could have predicted that one day I would more than likely find him in some emergency room, fighting for breath, nauseated, in a cold sweat, crushing pains tugging at his chest, showing all the signs of a heart attack.

* * *

168

If Hal Buckley was not my typical transplant patient, he was typical of the 1.5 million people who suffer heart attacks every year in this country. More than 300,000 of them die before they reach a hospital. Another 250,000 die after they arrive. One of them is dying every thirty-two seconds, despite everything that we can do for them.

More of them make it now than used to. Before the development of the coronary-care unit a quarter century ago, almost a third of those who lived long enough to reach a hospital died. But since the early 1960s, those units have made it possible to prevent many of the sudden heart stoppages from disastrous arrhythmias, the most dangerous being those irregular and ineffective heartbeats of the ventricle called ventricular fibrillation. And if we couldn't do it there, we had new drugs we could try and, as a last resort, electrical shocks to the chest that would regularize the heartbeat.

Twentieth-century care for a modern problem. Oh, people had always died of heart attacks, but not so abundantly as they did today. That's because in ages past, untreatable infectious diseases, injuries, violence, and malnutrition got them first. Now we lived long enough for stress, and high blood pressure, and cholesterol, and tobacco smoke, and atherosclerosis to do us in.

Most heart attacks result from atherosclerosis, or hardening of the arteries. We didn't even know about it until the middle of the last century, although we had known the role coronary arteries played in nourishing the heart since the great English physician William Harvey discovered them in the seventeenth century.

Not until 150 years later, when enough people were living into middle age and the effects of coronary-artery disease began to appear regularly, did another Englishman, William Heberden, observe the narrowing and clogging of those life-giving passageways and call it atherosclerosis. Around the turn of this century, a number of doctors began to suspect that this process led to the formation of clots that blocked the flow of blood and caused heart attacks.

It started in some people as early as childhood, this slow building up of calcium, fatty substances, a blood-clotting material named fibrin, waste products from the body's cells, and the soft, waxy cholesterol produced by the liver. This material circulated through the blood, sticking to the walls of the arteries, mixing together bit by bit, growing harder and harder until it became something called plaque.

In some people, the process accelerated in the third decade of their lives, fueled by the kind of food they ate and how they lived and what they did to their bodies. Smoking speeded it up; the more they smoked, the faster it developed. Fast-food joints and high-priced restaurants packaged a glut of cholesterol in junk meals and luscious-looking entrees and helped it grow apace. The televisions in their living rooms and bedrooms and studies and dens that kept them from walking or running or playing outside encouraged the process on its way. And the bosses who demanded overtime, the coworkers after their jobs, the spouses who cheated, the kids who rebelled, the IRS that wouldn't leave them alone, the traffic jams, the deadlines, the power lunches, all the stressful big deals of modern existence stewed the mixture, which slowly began to harden into the plaque encircling their hearts.

For most people, atherosclerosis begins in earnest during their fifties and sixties. But even though it is for the most part a disease of age, almost forty-five percent of those who died of heart attacks were under age sixty-five. That was because of guys like Hal Buckley. Guys like Hal Buckley practically poured the plaque directly into their arteries.

He was a Music City sales executive, a middle-aged man in a high-pressure business who smoked three and one-half packs of cigarettes a day, worked long weeks, often around the clock, ate bad food too fast on the way to somewhere else, made good money and put on weight, had no time for regular exercise and yet pushed himself hard when he did anything at all physical around the house.

He may not have had control over everything that caused his

heart trouble. No doubt about it, genes play a major role; he may have been born with a propensity for heart attacks. Many people are. He was a man, and his sex put him at greater risk. If he'd been black, or a diabetic, or genetically obese, there would have been little he could do to change the increased chances of his heart giving out on him. But he was none of those things, and there was plenty he could have done to cut down his risks.

He could have thrown away the cigarettes. They were making him four times more likely to suffer an attack, to die from it, and to die from it suddenly, within an hour. He could have eaten better, thrown out the salt and the junk food, exercised more and regularly, and found better ways to deal with the stress in his life. And he could have gone to a doctor and had his blood pressure and his cholesterol checked on a periodic basis.

Perhaps if Hal had done that, his doctor would have come into the examining room and strapped the rubber cuff called a sphygmomanometer around his upper right arm up against the big artery there and pumped air into the cuff and let it out slowly and felt for the pulse and discovered that Hal did not have the normal blood pressure of 120/80. Maybe Hal's systolic pressure, the first and larger number, would have been greater than 140 mm Hg; maybe his diastolic pressure would have been greater than 90 mm Hg. It would have meant that Hal was suffering from hypertension.

And the doctor would have recognized the high blood pressure as an all-important danger sign. Blood pressure is a measure of the force exerted by the blood against artery walls as the heart pumps it through the body. The doctor would have understood that Hal's heart was working harder than normal for some reason, that Hal's arteries were under great strain. If this had been going on for a long while or if it continued, it would enlarge Hal's heart, it would scar his arteries and make them less elastic, it would add to the buildup of plaque, speed up atherosclerosis, bring on a stroke, lead to a heart attack. But it could be treated if it was recognized, and with this treatment all these risks could be eliminated.

The doctor would have tested Hal's cholesterol, first with a simple pinprick blood sample from his thumb, then perhaps more elaborately. He would be looking for a cholesterol level of over 200 milligrams in Hal's blood. The normal level was around 150; anything over 240 milligrams doubled the risk of heart attack. Hal should have known what his cholesterol level was, just like he should have known what his blood pressure was. There are things he could have done by modifying his diet to lower his cholesterol level and decrease his risk for a heart attack.

And perhaps the doctor would have even ordered an arteriogram, most likely after an exercise treadmill test had been found to be abnormal. Hal would have checked briefly into the hospital for the test. Doctors would have run a thin plastic catheter through an artery in Hal's leg into each of the coronary arteries that fed his heart. They would have injected a liquid dye that lit up the arteries as they pumped blood to the heart muscle, making any obstruction clearly visible on high-speed x-ray movies.

If Hal's problem had been bad enough, he might have needed bypass surgery; more likely, the doctor first would have suggested medication, or a combination of medications, after a trial period to see what worked best. He would have put Hal on a salt-free diet low in saturated fats, warned him sternly to quit smoking, and prescribed an exercise regimen. But most of all, he would have made sure Hal understood the warning signs of a heart attack and what to do when they occurred.

He would have told Hal about angina pectoris, the chest pain that comes with myocardial ischemia, when the heart muscle, the myocardium, doesn't get the blood—and therefore the oxygen—it needs. He would have told him to watch out for any uncomfortable pressure, fullness, or squeezing in the center of the chest that lasted two minutes or more; stabbing pains in his shoulders, neck, and arms; any severe pain, especially one accompanied by dizziness, fainting, nausea, or shortness of breath.

But Hal had not done any of that. Vaguely aware at best that he fit the profile of a heart-attack victim, he told himself he had never been seriously ill a day in his life, he was at the peak of health, big, stronger than most of his friends, faster than them, virile, sexually active, competitive, hard driving, hard drinking, sharp. He didn't know, and didn't care to know, his cholesterol level. Sure, he was under a lot of stress, but it was stress he could handle, stress he was good at handling, stress that kept him honed and ready. Like ninety percent of those with hypertension, he was not aware he had it, if he in fact did. And like a million others, Hal could not recognize a heart attack when it walked up and kicked him in the chest.

He was at an all-night party that Saturday night having the time of his life with his friends, his buddies from work, and his neighbors, when the blood in his coronary arteries started to back up behind a clot. The clot itself might have formed on a crack in the fatty cholesterol deposits lining the walls of one of his arteries. He was drinking his scotch and waters and feeling good while his heart grew starved for oxygen. He was smoking cigarette after cigarette as one by one his heart cells shriveled up and died. He managed to drive himself home and was crawling into bed at three in the morning when enough blood cells had been damaged for the crushing chest pain to start. That night, Hal Buckley had experienced a mild myocardial infarction, a heart attack. He thought he just had a hangover and an upset stomach.

So did the local hospital when he checked in an hour later, saying that he had not had all that much to drink, but that he'd broken out into a sweat, started vomiting, and felt severe pains in his lower belly. The emergency-room personnel diagnosed indigestion, gave him pain killers, and sent him home with instructions to return if he didn't get better. Four hours later he was back, feeling much worse, dizzy, in severe pain, very short of breath. At first, since he had already been examined once, he was shunted aside, but then one of the physicians noticed him, stopped, asked him a few brief questions, then shouted, "Hey, this guy's had a heart attack."

Within five minutes, the doctors had inserted a tube in Hal's arm and infused him with a drug called tissue plasminogen activator, or TPA. A revolutionary new treatment born of the marriage between gene-splicing research and biotechnology, TPA and

173

similar drugs dissolved the blood clots that caused most heart attacks. In many, many cases these drugs prevented the permanent damage done by even mild myocardial infarctions. It was becoming standard therapy for most heart attacks.

Now Hal Buckley got his arteriogram, and the doctors found clots in all of his coronary arteries. It was clear that for Hal treatment had come too late. All three of the major arteries around Hal's heart had become narrowed and clogged by atherosclerosis.

The next day, the local hospital sent him thirty miles away to Vanderbilt. There, because he was not a candidate for bypass surgery, the cardiologists attempted a nonsurgical procedure called PTCA (percutaneous transluminal coronary angioplasty) in hopes of dilating the closed passageways around the heart. Doctors inserted a catheter into an artery in Hal's groin and guided it to one of the blocked coronary arteries. They passed a tiny balloon over the catheter and then inflated its tip at the point of blockage. They hoped to compress the plaque, enlarge the diameter of the blood vessel, and allow blood to flow more easily through the vessel.

It worked about seventy-five percent of the time. But in as many as half of the cases, the coronary artery collapsed back to its original narrow width within the first six months, forcing the patient to go through the procedure again and again or face an operation. The procedure has seen exponential growth in the past five years.

Surgeons tended to point to the common treatment failures, almost always arguing for the more definitive, although more invasive, procedure of bypass surgery. Cardiologists, who had to diagnose the underlying disease, perform the PTCA, and then evaluate its efficacy, hotly defended it. The debate raged, and only time would tell who was right. But in Hal's case, at least, the PTCA was no more successful than the TPA had been.

Hal's heart continued to deteriorate and water began to back up into his lungs, making it impossible for him to breathe on his own. He was put on a ventilator to support his lungs. His heart was severely, irreversibly damaged. To assist the pumping activity

174

of his weakened heart, the surgeons tried an intra-aortic balloon pump. Inserted in Hal's groin and up into his aorta, close to his heart, the balloon expanded and collapsed in synchrony with the relaxation and contraction of the heart, taking over about twenty percent of the heart's pumping function. It kept him alive long enough for the cardiologists to tell Hal that every conventional treatment known to mankind had been tried and had failed. Long enough to warn him that—without a heart transplant—he would die.

I met him for the first time that night.

Six weeks later, Hal was sitting with his wife, Pam, in one of my examining rooms. He was trim and ruddy, with close-cropped sandy hair, dressed in a thousand dollars' worth of casual clothes, watching me with intelligent, ironic eyes, turning as I walked in, and saying in his quick, hip, aggressive way, "OK, Frist, when do I go back to work?"

"Well, first we have to make sure you're well. Get a biopsy today and see—"

"I'm fine. I feel great. I'm going a little stir-crazy, but otherwise—"

"You may feel fine, Hal, but that doesn't mean a thing. It can change like that." I snapped my fingers. "You have to get used to the idea that you can't rely solely on the way you feel, like you used to, to know entirely how well you're doing. That's why we have all these precautions, make you come in and visit us on a regular basis, why we run all these sophisticated tests."

Hal was shaking his head and smiling. When I looked at Pam, she quickly glanced away.

"Dr. Frist, Dr. Frist," Hal said. "You don't have to give me the patient pep talk. I understand all that. And I'm being a good boy: taking all my medicines, keeping track of my blood pressure, right, Pam?"

Pam turned back from the window and said to me pointedly, "He's taking all his medicines."

"I know it's your job," Hal said. "And I admire you for it.

175

You're good at it. I've looked into this. You are a very capable man and you are building an advanced program here. I can look around and see that you're taking chances other programs don't take, helping people they wouldn't select. So I know you're more humanistic, but you're also more confident. You figure you can keep your success rate—"

"Hal—," I said. From the moment Hal had opened his eyes after surgery, his treatment had been a chess game between the two of us, one I had resigned myself to playing six weeks ago. I knew his flattery was just another move, a tricky gambit.

"No, no," he said, holding up his index finger. "Let me finish. No matter how good you are, Dr. Frist, the statistics are against me. How long have I got, really? Five good years, ten at the most, a little more if I'm lucky? Well, I'm capable and confident, too, but I'm in sales. You come from money, so you can't understand exactly what that means. Yes, my insurance covered the operation, and yes, it's going to cover the medicine, but it's only going to go up to a million, and I'll be well beyond that before I'm done."

"Hal—"

There was no stopping him. "Oh, they say they'll take me back at work, but they aren't stupid. They'll be looking for a way to get rid of me. And in sales, you've got to produce. I've got to get back, do my job, protect myself with a good record, and make sure in the six or seven years left I put enough away to last Pam after I'm gone and to educate my kids."

He just couldn't help it, I thought. For him all conversation was, and always had been, a contest. It was his nature. But now the game had turned deadly, and still he felt compelled to play it. He couldn't win and survive. I had to win if he was going live.

"Hal, those statistics you're reading are based on treatment regimens that are outdated. And if I gave you today's numbers, in six months they'd be out of date. Right now transplantation has as good long-term treatment results as bypass surgery, better than all standard therapies for cancer, and it's getting better. If you go back to work before you're ready, you'll die, and I'm not going to let that happen no matter what you say. If you lose your job, I'll pay for the rest of the treatment personally, out of my own pocket if I have to. But I'm the one who decides when you are ready."

Check. Hal looked at me, shrugged, said, "You're the doctor." And I touched his hand, shrugged, and said, "All right! I thought you'd never get that straight. Now get on out of here, find Jan, and go have your biopsy. We'll talk about work when I see the results."

I walked over and sat in a swivel chair near the medicine cabinet and sink as the two of them got up to leave. "Hal," I said, just as they got to the door, "why don't you go on and let Pam stay here and talk to me for a minute."

"What's up?" he said.

"Nothing," I said. "I just need to talk to her so the two of us can figure out some way to make you behave."

His smile looked forced. Jan was right, something was going on between them.

"Never happen," he said. Then to her, "Don't let his boyish charm and his conventional good looks fool you."

When he had gone, I went right to the point. "Pam, what's happening with you two?"

She didn't answer right away. She tried to say something and choked up, tears welling in her eyes. I told her to sit down, guided her to the examination table, and put my hand on her shoulder.

"Take your time," I said.

She starting sobbing, looked away, then cried freely in big heaves. After a while the story came out.

"Dr. Frist, he hasn't been himself since surgery. He has violent temper tantrums. He won't let me see his medicines. I mean he hides them from me. He won't tell me what he's supposed to take. He won't talk to his family. He fights with his brother. He yells at me all the time. And at the girls."

"Does he scare you?"

She nodded her head.

"This is hard for me to ask," I said. "But did he do these things before, I mean before his operation? Has he ever physically abused you?"

She shook her head.

"He always had a quick temper. But he's not himself. It's like he's, I don't know, psychotic or something. Our oldest daughter, Debra—she's seventeen—she's threatening to leave."

I talked to Pam for a long time that afternoon. I calmed her down and told her that Hal was not psychotic, that he was going through an exaggerated form of the adjustment problems we saw in most of our patients. I told her the side effects of his medicine might be causing some of his erratic behavior. I explained that Hal was going through a period of denial, that he could not admit that he was a transplant recipient, that he was testing everything and everyone around him.

And I told her not to worry.

I would handle everything. I would talk to Hal, I would get him an appointment today with our team psychiatrist, Dr. Scott West, who followed all our transplant patients. Later on, maybe, it would help if she attended sessions with Hal, but we'd leave it up to Dr. West.

After she had gone, I held a conference with Jan and Walter and Janie Webb, the social worker, and we went over essentially the same points. We discussed Hal's medication and decided, pending the results of today's biopsy, to lower his dosages, especially of the steroid prednisone. Its side effects could resemble a mild psychosis. Jan got Dr. West on the phone for me, and I described for him what was going on. We discussed the possibility of Hal going back to work, at least part time.

"I'll have to talk to him, of course," West said. "But on the face of it, it might not be a bad idea."

After I had put the receiver down, I turned to Jan.

"You know what strikes me?" I said. "Hal's right. I mean he's confused, he's angry, he can't think straight, but we are about to do just what he suggested we do: cut back his prednisone and send him back to work."

"This really bothers you, doesn't it?" Jan said.

"You mean that he's right or that he's such a mental mess?"

178

"About his family. How he's treating them."

"Oh," I said, "sure. I'm not overly worried at this point. It's serious, but we'll get him back on track. He's a smart man, self-aware. With a little help. . . . But it's his normal personality I worry about. Once he's up and running, I bet it won't be two weeks before he's putting in sixty hours again, working around the clock. Checkmate."

"What?"

"Nothing," I said. "It's all part of the game."

Jan gave me an odd look. "Didn't you say Hal reminded you of certain surgeons you knew?" she said with a wicked grin.

4

Jan and I walked into examining room five. When I saw Hugh Trigg waiting with his wife, I realized how truly mentally unprepared Hal Buckley had been to receive a transplant. He had not had the years of knowing he was sick, of wandering from one specialist to the next as his condition grew worse, of finally being told he needed a new heart, of going home and thinking it over and slowly beginning to imagine himself as a transplant recipient. He had not had the descriptive talks, the careful walking through of the process, the answering of every question that Jan and I were about to provide Hugh Trigg. True, I had discussed transplantation with Hal when I first met him in the hospital. I had explained everything just as I would now to Trigg, just as I did to each new patient. But Hal had been in the middle of the biggest crisis of his life, with a ventilator supporting his lungs and a balloon pump assisting his heart, full of pain killers, numbed by all that had happened to him. He simply couldn't take it all in.

Most of all, I thought rather grimly, Hal hadn't gone through the long agonizing wait for a donor organ that Hugh Trigg was about to experience. Hal had not worried about how high his name was on the list, had not wondered who around him was getting a heart before him and why, had not suffered through false starts, like Jimmy Moore waiting anxiously for us to check out a donor and then having us say no go. And there was always the distinct possibility that a heart could not be found in time.

While that wait was terrible, it did teach them quite viscerally how privileged, how really lucky they were. I thought particularly of Charles Mullins, one of my first transplant patients at Vanderbilt, a sweet man in his fifties. He still cried every time he told the story about his close friend, a traffic controller at the Crossville

180

airport, who had been on duty in the tower the night Walter Merrill, white knuckles gripping knocking knees, came flying back into town in a Lear jet with Mullins's new heart in an Igloo cooler on the luxurious seat beside him.

Over Crossville, the intercom in the plane had crackled, and a voice identified itself as center control.

"Are you carrying a human heart?" the voice asked.

The pilot, puzzled, said yes he was, and he heard a round of cheers go up in the tower. "Now you take good care of that heart," the voice said. "It's for a buddy of ours."

And the group in the tower had tracked the Lear jet all the way into Nashville, their eyes glued to the lifesaving little blip on their radar screen.

No, I thought, Hal Buckley had none of that. His friends and acquaintances had been shocked to hear that so robust a fellow had had a transplant, and Hal clung to their image of him. Understandably enough, he blamed the local hospital that had misdiagnosed his trouble. He perpetuated in his own mind the myth that he had been incredibly healthy before the accident of his heart attack. It came out now in his adjustment problems, his anger, his frustration, his anxiety to get back to work.

Hugh Trigg could entertain no such illusions. I had seen him the first time a year before, but the cardiomyopathy that was bloating his heart had not yet caused sufficient damage for me to list him. I had explained that he had a seventy percent chance of making it through the next two years. I sent him home to get sicker. It was always hard to predict how fast someone would deteriorate, how long one would live without a transplant. We did not want to transplant people too early, especially given the shortage of organs. But it was equally bad waiting too long, having a patient die who could have lived with a transplant.

The disease inexorably worked its damage on Hugh's heart, and now he was back, a big, dark-haired man in a wheel chair, a 6'5" fellow so weak he couldn't walk across the room without exhausting himself. Had I waited too long?

"You've got a huge heart," I said, "and it's not pumping very

181

well. That's why you feel so terrible and are always so weak, why you look so much worse than the last time."

Hugh's wife, a prim woman in her forties, looked at me expectantly and said with something approaching hope, "Do his cath pressures indicate that the transplant should be moved ahead—quickly?"

"Well," I said, looking down at the file on my lap as I sat up close to Hugh on the examining table, touching him lightly, reassuringly, on the arm. "His blood pressure and the other tests and the x-rays all indicate that if we wait too much longer it won't be just his heart. His lungs, too, will be irreversibly damaged. The pulmonary-artery pressure, the pressure in your lung arteries, is 60/40 and that's why you have some swelling in your feet and feel bloated all the time. Your heart is pumping so poorly that fluid is accumulating in your lungs, making it hard to breathe." I gave his arm a squeeze. "These lung pressures are fifty percent higher than they should be. The cardiac output for a man your size— that's the amount of blood your heart can pump out to your body in a minute—is about half of what it should be. And that's why you don't feel good." I patted him on his shoulder. "Your body's just not getting enough blood."

I took a breath, stood up, stepped back, crossed my arms, and looked him in the eye. "So how do things work overall from here?" I said. "I must tell you—even as you know—we have problems getting donors. We don't have any more problems at Vanderbilt than they do anywhere else, but our problem is bad. Do you by chance know your blood type?"

"A-positive."

"A-positive," I repeated. "Well, it could be anywhere from a week or two weeks to as long as six months or a year. I just can't—"

"Does he have that much time?" his wife asked, shooting me a glance.

"I can't tell you that, I'm sorry. What I do know is that your pulmonary pressures are bad enough that we should list you immediately and get this matter taken care of. I know you feel that way."

182

"I sure do," Hugh said.

"Now, how things work logistically. Basically, I'll get you listed tonight. That means you are placed on a nationwide computer network and given a status based on your size, blood type, how sick you are, and how long you have been waiting. When a donor becomes available, probably somewhere within seven or eight hundred miles, I will call you on the telephone. Because you are so big and because your pulmonary artery pressures are high, we will need to find a big heart for you. That means we cannot take just any donor; in fact we can't use a woman's heart because it would simply not be powerful enough. Unfortunately this size requirement is going to cut down on the number of potential donors out there for you."

Hugh stared blankly at his wife.

"Jan will ask Faye, our secretary, to get you a beeper," I said, "so we can get in touch with you twenty-four hours a day. It may take a week, maybe two, to get the beeper, but after that you'll have it with you, so that the instant a donor heart becomes available I can call you up and say, 'Hi, there, Hugh. Say, why don't you mosey on down to the hospital.' "

When I had them smiling, I went on. "No. I'll call you, tell you to get down here as quickly as you can, and you'll be able to do that. You'll get to Vanderbilt, and at that point things will move very quickly, and I'll meet you in the operating room and—poof— that's it. You'll be a new man. You won't see a lot of other doctors, just me primarily, and Dr. Merrill, and Jan here."

"How long does the surgery last?" Mrs. Trigg asked, and I smiled. She was the one who would wait anxiously through the operation.

"It really depends on the timing and location of the donor," I said. "It takes a lot of organization to get us up in those airplanes, flying around, picking up those hearts, and getting them back here in time, while we get you all ready for the operation here. We never take your old heart out, though, till we're sure about the new one and we have it in the room there with you."

"Who gets the donor heart?" she asked.

"I do. Or Dr. Merrill."

"Not many people know how to do that, do they?" I knew she was asking for reassurance that we did know exactly how to do it.

"Not many," I said. "But the real reason we go get the hearts ourselves is so we'll know exactly how it has been handled, that it was taken with an extra degree of care. It is all a system, and I can promise you that we've got that system down pat here."

"How long will I stay in the hospital?" Trigg asked. He was the one who would wait anxiously through the recovery.

"Anywhere from two to six weeks. Almost everybody has some rejection, as I explained to you earlier. And just about everybody has some infection at some point after the operation." I always told every patient to expect these two complications as normal events after transplantation. They both occurred frequently, and it was important for a patient not to interpret these problems as setbacks after surgery.

"But our role in this whole scenario—my personal as well as professional contract with you, and Dr. Merrill's contract, and Jan's—is to walk you through this whole process a step at a time." When a patient thinks about the whole process of transplantation, it is overwhelming; it would be for anybody. By breaking the entire process into many little steps, a series of little challenges, it becomes more tolerable and comprehensible.

"We'll get you through the surgery. Like I said, you'll have some rejection and infection, but we'll get you through that, too. We'll get you through each of the things that come up. Day by day you'll meet a new challenge. But I know this backwards and forwards, and I know we'll get you through it. There will be ups and downs. It will be discouraging at times. You'll get upset with me at times, especially when I march you through tests that may seem unnecessary. I can promise you that at some point, you will be depressed. Maybe you won't recover as fast as we would like; if you don't, I'll tell you so. When we are dealing with issues of life and death, issues related to your welfare, I have always found it best to lay all the cards on the table, no secrets. I'll shoot straight with you from the outset. And that's about it. We'll get you through this just fine."

"Will I still feel bad after surgery?"

"You sure will," I laughed. "Surgery is kind of like getting hit by a truck."

Hugh Trigg gulped, "You said you'd shoot straight."

"But you'll get through it," I said. "And you'll feel bad for a while. And then one day, maybe a week after the operation or maybe a month, you'll suddenly realize Hey, I feel OK. I feel pretty good. You've been sick for so long, it'll take you a while to get used to feeling normal again."

"What about this, Dr. Frist?" Mrs. Trigg said. I looked down at what she was holding out to me—an issue of *Time* magazine with a picture of the Jarvik-7, the controversial artificial heart used by Dr. William DeVries in Salt Lake City. "Are you familiar with it?"

"Yes, I am," I said. "That's called the Jarvik heart, and it's an interesting device that can be very useful. A lot of people ask about it because it's gotten so much publicity in the last few years. But, you know, we are not using it here. It is not very good as a permanent heart, but it's currently being used to support people who are waiting for a transplant once their own heart gives out completely. We have a different device, much better than this one, one we have a lot more experience with. But here, Jan why don't you take over for a minute? I'm just going to step into my office and pick up something and show you what I'm talking about."

Jan moved in very smoothly as I stepped out the door, saying to Hugh, "Are you feeling worse than when I saw you in the hospital room? You look like you are feeling weaker, but I am glad your spirits are still high. Let me go over everything in a little more detail. And, please, feel free to ask any questions."

From the beginning, artificial hearts meant big trouble. An early version of such a device had led to the final and now-famous split between Denton Cooley and his erstwhile mentor, the even more renowned Michael DeBakey. DeBakey had been working on an artificial heart for a number of years with one of his technicians. Some claimed it was a way to gain back the glory his talented former "student" Cooley had stolen from him by jumping so fully onto the ill-starred heart-transplant bandwagon of the late 1960s.

But once again, Cooley jumped the gun on DeBakey. While DeBakey was off on one of his many trips to Washington, D.C., in April 1969, Cooley persuaded—his detractors thought the word *browbeat* would be more appropriate—a terminally ill patient to let him implant the artificial heart as a bridge to transplantation until a donor became available.

The results were disastrous. The patient fared very badly indeed, living sixty-eight hours before a donor became available and Cooley removed the device, then dying about twenty hours after that. DeBakey was furious, accused Cooley of theft, and started a campaign against Cooley that led to a full-scale governmental investigation of his ethics. And the patient's wife, angry with Cooley for allegedly misinforming her and her husband about the nature of the treatment, sued him for malpractice. The rift between DeBakey, The Texas Tornado, and Cooley, dubbed Mr. Wonderful, has continued to this day.

Branded as glory-hunting experimentation, artificial hearts suffered a greater eclipse than even heart transplants until a group of doctors led by William DeVries, then at the University of Utah, successfully implanted the Jarvik-7 in Barney Clark in 1982. Four others followed. All but two of the patients died within a few days or months, but two continued to live even after DeVries moved to Louisville where Humana promised him the funds to continue his work.

There were problems. William Schroeder, one of the two living patients, had suffered a series of strokes. After a year and a half on the device, he had essentially become unresponsive. Murray Haydon, the other recipient, was still on a respirator more than a year after his surgery. The Jarvik heart was a pneumatic device. Compressed air from a huge machine ran through large tubes running straight to the mechanical heart in the patient's chest. Fueled by the compressor, the mechanical heart pumped the blood through the body. The pump of course couldn't be turned off, and the patient was chained to it, doomed to this unwieldy umbilical cord for the rest of his life or until a donor

186

heart could be found. Infections formed readily around the tubes, and blood clots had a tendency to form in the little pools of blood that backed up in corners of the artificial heart's various chambers.

At that point, DeVries was the only doctor in America with Food and Drug Administration approval to do permanent artificial implants, but criticism of his mechanical hearts, even as bridges to transplantation, was growing. Foremost among those critics was Norman Shumway. Ten times as much money had been spent on the Jarvik as had been spent on transplantation, and that irritated Shumway. He thought Humana was merely after publicity, touting the Jarvik so the company could get more customers for other kinds of surgery. And he thought the Jarvik was a failure because of the threat of blood clotting.

I could just see his ice-blue eyes flash as he waxed eloquent on the subject. "I get angry when they use the thing as a bridge. Once you're on the Jarvik, you're in such jeopardy—the damn thing is really very dangerous—you go right up to the top of the waiting list. And all that does is make the shortage of donors worse. The guy in the next bed, who's equally deserving, doesn't have a chance. The way it's worked out, it's sort of a gimmick to get a heart.

"These engineers come to you and they say, 'Now look, Doc, the heart's just a pump, right? And we can make you any kind of pump.'" Then his eyebrows would go up and he'd appear incredulous. "That's stupid. We don't even have a truly satisfactory heart valve, and the Jarvik's got four of them. We can get by in blood-vessel surgery by putting in plastic tubes because they just lie there and don't do anything. It's when everything starts to move that you run into problems.

"To be anywhere comparable to a transplant, a mechanical heart has to be totally implantable and driven by a inexhaustible source. We don't have anything like that. If we did, we'd put it in our automobiles first, then maybe our refrigerators, and finally, maybe, in our artificial hearts."

And Phil Oyer listened to him, went back to his computers and his lab, put his problem-solving mind to work. With Peer Portner, an inventor and scientist from a company called Novacor, he began to perfect a type of mechanical heart called a left-ventricular assist device. A few years, a lot of research, and $32 million in government and venture-capital funds later, a model of the LVAD sat in my office on the shelf behind my desk. Its elegant hollow ceramic chamber fit snugly in the palm of my hand as I picked it up to take it in and show the Triggs.

While I was gone, Hugh and his wife bombarded Jan with questions. After she had explained how we screened donors and discussed how we make sure the donor heart is a good match, Hugh asked, "What about AIDS? Is that a threat?"

"We screen the donors for AIDS, and we exclude potential donors who are at high risk, like intravenous drug users," Jan said.

"I'll need some blood during surgery, won't I?" he pushed. "Why don't I give my own blood?"

"Well," Jan said, "you can't give your own blood because of your severe heart condition. That's not a good idea. But if you want to have family or friends give blood specifically for you, we can arrange that. Of course, they must be the same blood type. Fresh blood is only good for forty-two days, and if you are waiting for a long while it can expire. We never let that happen; we transfer it to someone who needs it before it does. Probably what we would do for you is freeze the blood; that way it can be held in storage for a long while, available to be thawed when we need it. You know, receiving blood is a type of transplant as well."

"My brother would do it," Hugh said. "He's back home in Virginia."

"That's a problem," Jan said. "They have to go to the Red Cross to donate, so you need somebody here. And it has to be somebody local. If you want to do this, there is some paperwork, and Dr. Frist has to sign a waiver saying you are on your own to get the blood. But let me tell you this: I know you've heard some horror stories about the Red Cross and contaminated blood, but we've done some studies, statistical studies, comparing volunteer blood obtained and screened by the blood bank here in Nashville with donor-directed blood like we were discussing. We have found absolutely no difference in the incidence of hepatitis or AIDS, which these days is very, very small anyway."

"What's the chance of me not getting a donor before it's too late? Does that happen much?"

"That has happened," Jan said. "I can't really give you numbers. I don't really know. We've had some people die waiting, and that's discouraging. We hate to see it, and we are going to do everything we can to make certain we get one for you. That's why it's important that if you start getting even sicker that we know about it, because that changes your severity of illness rating and we adjust your status on the computer list."

"Where will he be on the list?" asked Mrs. Trigg.

"We have several people who are waiting, but they are different blood types and different sizes. The way it works right now is that we rate you according to need. Need is determined by where you are, whether you are at home or the hospital—basically, how sick you are. And, of course, blood type and body size."

"So he won't be at the top of the list because he's at home?"

"That's right," Jan said. "But there are so many factors involved."

"Can't you just check him into the hospital?"

"We can't do that."

"Why not?"

"You can't really look at it that way. Even if he is here in the hospital, and somebody else is sicker—in the ICU, for example—then their need is greater, and we have to take them first, all things being equal. But they never are. We have to match body size and blood type first. It's not fair to yourself to start thinking, 'Oh, he's number five,' because it never works out like that."

"I'm getting weaker," Hugh said.

When I came back into the room, Jan was explaining what would happen once they got the call. "Very occasionally we have a patient come in when we thought we had a good donor heart and then something showed up that made us think we shouldn't go ahead. We had one patient go as far as the OR. It's always disappointing and hard because you get—you think, Gosh, it's finally here, you know, and sort of get psyched up for it. But in the vast majority of cases we proceed with the transplant. What I've found from talking to patients and families is that it's more likely you will get cold feet. People are relieved when we call up and say it looks like we have a possible donor, and they get here and things are moving very fast, and they say, 'Whoa. Wait. Let me out.' People are excited, but they are also very scared. That's normal. We understand it. We have a guy here today, walking around big as life who at first just said 'No way.' "

Jan paused and looked at me. I handed the LVAD to Mrs. Trigg, but I aimed my remarks at Hugh. "I guess this is something we need to talk about." As I addressed him it became obvious to me that he was tiring so much easier than the rest of us.

"We need to think about, potentially, if you go downhill and we have to bring you back to the hospital, it might be that we need to consider using this artificial heart."

I showed them the small, symmetrical LVAD and the two long half-inch wide tubes.

"These attach to the device, and we put this tube here right into the left side of your heart at the bottom. This one here we attach at the top to your aorta. We don't take your old heart out, just place this beside it, sort of piggyback. The whole thing goes inside, with just this one thin wire coming out.

"It runs by electricity. It's the only one that does. We are working on one that has a power source, about the size of a cigarette pack, which we attach to a belt surgically implanted beneath the skin around your waist. With that power pack we could charge up the heart so you wouldn't have to be plugged into a machine all the time; you could get out of bed, walk around, take a shower. That model will be totally implantable, so even the wire won't be sticking out. We tested it on a sheep for the first time six weeks ago, and it works.

"We're one of six centers in the country the FDA allows to use this device. It's purely investigational, but we've used it in over two hundred animals, and it works well. We've used it in about twenty-two people. We have used it as a bridge to transplantation, and the results are good. There can be side effects, but nothing like that Jarvik heart in the magazine there, which has a tendency to cause strokes, bleeding, and infection. It's not anywhere near as experimental or investigational as that. We've been working on it since 1974 and over $30 million has gone into its development. It's the only one designed for total implantation, the only one that has a truly implantable, fully integrated control system."

"Thirty million dollars!" Hugh said. "Do I have to pay in cash?"

"The money to develop it came from the National Institutes of Health and from venture-capital money placed into a private company called Novacor."

"It's light," said Mrs. Trigg.

"About a pound and a half."

"How does it work?"

"Well, as I said, we implant it next to the heart. With most patients with heart trouble, like you, it's really their left ventricle—the heart's main pumping chamber—that's critical. This is a left-ventricular assist device, meaning it is attached to the ventricle and takes the outflow of blood through this tube, here, and allows the ventricle to rest.

"The blood flows into the device here from the ventricle, circulates like this, then goes through an outflow valve here up into the aorta—the main blood vessel coming off the heart—meanwhile flooding all the vital organs with blood, taking them the nutrients and oxygen they need. See these little pusher plates? They move the blood along. It's symmetrical, so you don't have a lot of pulsation, like you do with the other devices. You don't have any little pockets where blood can build up, like the Jarvik. And you don't have those huge pneumatic tubes sticking out of your chest.

"The LVAD can take over the total cardiac output and, in

191

effect, your own left ventricle does not need to beat at all. It can be dead, or just an empty, static conduit, and this device will take over, pump your blood all through your body. We're using it mainly now as a bridge to transplantation. That's what we might need to use it for in your case. We can talk about it more when the time comes, *if* the time comes."

I was trying not to act like a kid with his favorite toy. There would be so many possibilities when the LVAD was perfected. I had used the LVAD only once since coming to Vanderbilt, on Richard Gibson. He had come into the hospital suffering from massive heart failure even worse than Hal Buckley's, but there had been no matching heart awaiting his arrival. He would have died right there if his wife had not agreed to use the mechanical heart.

As with the heart-lung transplant, I had trained the surgical team to implant the LVAD using sheep in the lab, and there was a lot of excitement when Mrs. Gibson agreed to give the device a try. And the excitement had grown as we got Gibson into the OR, made the long incision all the way down to his abdomen, tucked the little piece of ceramic up under his abdominal wall, and let the LVAD take over, the click, click, click of its pusher plates replacing the rhythmic thumping of his heart.

Gibson was much too sick to list before he got the LVAD, but four days later he had recovered enough that we could begin the process of looking for a donor. For thirty-two days he lay in the bed as we waited for a heart to become available, his ECG absolutely flat because his heart wasn't beating, the clicking of the LVAD signaling that blood was pumping through his body. Mrs. Gibson and the children would go in and talk to him, anxiously explaining what they had done, trying to gauge his reaction by the look in his eyes as they glanced back and forth.

And then words began to return to him, and slowly the family became adept at understanding what he was trying to say through the contorted syntax of his illness. He let them know they had made the right decision. I was sure we were going to make it, and then as if to prove me right a call came from up

North saying the computers had come up with a match. The donor heart was not perfect—it had been allowed to lie fallow for too long after brain death before the body, languishing in the hospital room, was put on a respirator—but I was afraid it was the best we were going to get.

Richard Gibson died a few hours after transplant surgery. As with everything in this field, any number of explanations might have accounted for his death. Gibson's other organs may have been too damaged by his initial heart attack to survive even with a perfect heart, but he could not in that event have carried on much longer as he was. It sounds cold, but I took a grim satisfaction in the fact that at least the LVAD had performed perfectly in its role as a bridge to transplantation.

The press, of course, much interested in the operation because no one else in the region was using the artificial heart, confused the issues, blaming what was essentially a donor-shortage problem on the LVAD itself. And that was the problem with the artificial heart's controversial history. There was the danger that we would throw out the baby with the bath water, that responding to negative public feelings, the government would cut off funding for all mechanical devices, even one so promising as this.

I had no way of knowing, then, that the government would do just that within six months, that the NIH would stop much of its research on the Jarvik and all other artificial hearts except for the Novacor LVAD. That day, holding clinic, sitting there with the Triggs, watching the two of them stare at the device and try to imagine it somehow inside Hugh Trigg's body, I just hoped we would have time to perfect it before the public and the government gave up. The LVAD, I knew, could eventually help alleviate the donor problem. There are as many as ten thousand people a year who could benefit from such a device once it is perfected, people who now have no alternative. We will never have that many human donor hearts to transplant, so the only way to fill the gap is to develop a workable and safe artificial device.

And I found myself wondering if Hugh Trigg would actually

make it. A-positive was not all that hard a match, he was sick enough to place high on the list, and he had a good chance of lasting long enough for us to find a match. But it was out of my control. We could only wait—and pray.

He was much better off than the poor devil I had seen next door at the Veterans Administration Hospital that morning. Billy Jones was an indigent man, barely hanging onto life with a series of short-term, part-time jobs as a dishwasher and a fry cook even before his heart gave out on him from years of poverty and hard living. He was Hal Buckley's age, forty-three. But he looked eighty.

The opposite of Hugh the first time I had seen him, Billy was too sick to list right now. He had congestive heart failure—a condition that occurs from damage to the heart muscle as a result of such things as high blood pressure, heart attacks, atherosclerosis, a congenital heart defect, rheumatic fever, pressure on the heart from lung disease, any number of things. His heart simply lacked the strength to keep his blood circulating, causing his ankles and legs to swell and his breathing to become difficult. He also had diabetes.

Even if the VA nursed him back to a condition I could work with in the system, I didn't know that I would list him. He was so down and out, so alone, so shiftless. With the diabetes and with no one to help him through his lifelong post-op course, I might well be wasting a heart. Despair clung to every answer he gave when I interviewed him.

As Jan stepped in and talked to the Triggs about the operation itself, demystifying the process of explaining everything from the incision to the final stitch, I could hear Billy's lonesome voice rattling about in my head.

"You work here?" he had asked, distrust staring from the sunken eyes in his skull of a face when I had introduced myself.

"I work at Vanderbilt," I said. "And at the VA here, sometimes. I work both places."

He was staring blankly.

"Anyway," I went on, "they've asked me to come by and see

you. Talk to you a little bit about your history and try to decide what's best overall."

"The first thing is that I don't have a history," he said.

"What were you doing before all this happened?"

"Just my job."

"And what's that? What do you do?"

"I'm a cook. Was a cook."

"So you cook. And who do you live with?"

"Myself."

"Do you have an apartment? I mean, now. Still. Since you've been in the hospital."

"Yeah," he lied.

"Do you have a family?"

A crafty expression crept over his face, and for the first time he seemed truly alive. "I want to live with my sister."

"Tell me what happened to you," I said. "When did—"

"First of December," he said, shutting his mouth tight. I waited.

"You were cooking?"

"No. I come in one night and I noticed my feet had begin to swell. Next thing it goes up through my leg. Through my waist. So it's up, it's down, and it's swelling."

"How much do you weigh?"

"A hundred pounds."

"How much did you weigh a year ago?"

"Oh, about 160 pounds."

"So you lost some weight. I thought cooks were supposed to eat a lot."

"They are," he said. "But you know you get tired."

"Do you drink alcohol? Did you ever?"

"Never have."

"What about smoking?"

"Yeah, I smoked a little."

"Do you smoke now? When did you stop?"

"I stopped . . . five years. Beer, whiskey, cigarettes, I stopped it all. Five years ago, I swear."

"How'd you stop?"

"Just threw 'em away."

"All of a sudden one day? Why?"

"Well, I just decided it was wasted money. The beer and the alcohol, I just threw them away."

"So let me tell you," I said. "I'm not sure what we're going to do. They're going to do a heart catheterization. When are they going to do that? Did they say?"

No answer.

"They'll probably do that early next week," I said. "They've asked me to come and talk to you. There are no medicines that will make your heart better. Do you understand? They got the fluid off, but your heart's not working. The only therapy we have now is a heart transplant. Have they talked to you about it?"

Finally, he answered. "A little."

"What do you think about transplantation?"

"It would be all right if I could afford it."

"Money aside, what do you—"

"It's expensive, isn't it?"

"Let's not talk about the expense right now. We can worry about that later. Money aside, what do you think about a transplant?"

"What do you think?"

"I think for people who need it, it's pretty good."

"Well, that's kind of what I thought. Trouble is finding one."

"Finding what?"

"A donor."

"Finding a donor," I said. "How do you know about that?"

"You got to have a donor to have one."

You got to have a donor to have one. Billy's whiskey voice, filled with sadness, stayed with me as I gave him my card, told him to call me if he needed anything, and said I'd be back. I walked out of his room and out of the VA, its halls smelling of stale smoke, back to the spotless halls and antiseptic cleanliness of Vanderbilt fifty yards and a world away. You got to have a donor to have one.

196

Thinking about Billy as I sat in the room with the Triggs, I had lost the thread of the conversation. Mrs. Trigg was looking at me oddly, as if she had seen something in my face, my expression, she had not expected.

"Dr. Frist?" she said.

She did not know me well enough to ask me what I was thinking about, so instead she meekly handed me the mechanical heart she had been holding all this time.

5

Al Moore could remember vividly the first time he had ever felt it. He was thirty, backpacking on a weekend camping trip in the Smoky Mountains. It was one of those crisp, cool, crystal-clear autumn days, when the fiery leaves glowed in the sun as if the trees had been backlit for a movie. He thought it was the smoking and swore he'd cut down. Then one morning he got out of his car and walked up the steps to the Metro Courthouse where he was trying a case, and suddenly the shortness of breath was back. Only this time, his heart was racing too. Soon he would feel it as he dug postholes for his new fence, or washed the car, even as he played with his daughter. Before long, walking the three blocks from his house to his office was like taking a safari.

The first visit to Vanderbilt came about casually. One of the guys at the office had a wife who was a pediatrician. They made an appointment for him to see Dr. Craig Heim, with whom she was taking a course. Al went in order not to embarrass them, and he came out three days later knowing a new word: *cardiomyopathy.* Somewhere, somehow, a virus had gotten into his heart, and he was in trouble. But Heim and his colleagues had said they thought he would be OK if they put him on those drugs. He would never run in the Olympics, but he would be able to get by.

And he was OK for a while. He put in his seventy-hour weeks, tried a big case up in Kentucky, went in for his checkups, got by. Then he got back from Kentucky one Friday afternoon and there was a message from Dr. Heim that said "Call immediately."

"You said to call?" Al asked when the operator had tracked down Dr. Heim.

"Al. Yes. We noticed that you're having some ventricular

198

arrhythmia and we don't—it's very dangerous. You need to get over here right away."

"Fine, Craig," Al said. "I'll come, let me check my calendar here. How's Monday? No, actually Tuesday would be better if that's—"

"No, Al. I'm talking about right now."

This time Dr. Heim drew him a picture of his heart. When he started sketching, Al knew things were bad. The specialist showed him how his heart was turning into scar tissue. He called it a restrictive cardiomyopathy. He explained that Al had a good squeezing heart, but it didn't get enough blood, so it was becoming stiff and hard, unlike the floppy and weak hearts of the others.

"Other what?" Al asked.

"Other people who need a heart transplant," Dr. Heim said.

The first thing he worried about was the money. But then he found out that insurance at his law firm would cover it. The next thing he worried about was seeing his daughter Heather grow up. He had seen Barney Clark on TV—like so many, he confused transplants with artificial hearts—and he thought none of them worked very well. That you always had blood clots and strokes or lived like a vegetable. So who would take care of his family? He sat around and thought about every time he had a cigarette, every fat, juicy steak he had ever eaten, every night he had stayed out too late and drunk too much. His uncle, a graduate of Yale Divinity School and pastor at Woodland Hills, helped him out, talking about the hereafter and life and death and finding him a few good books to read.

He looked into transplant programs, checked out Birmingham, Houston, and Stanford, and had decided on the last until he heard about this new surgeon at Vanderbilt who came from California. The day we met, Al Moore said to me, "I got up this morning to come down here and I said to myself, 'Well, hell, we can either make the best of this or I can go jump off a bridge this afternoon.' Let's make the best of it."

And we did. It wasn't easy. We tried him on an investiga-

199

tional drug named flecainide to keep the blood flowing until we found him a heart. Instead, Al went into shock. Once we got him better and back out of the hospital, he and his wife separated. She had difficulty dealing with his disease, the way he tells it. She had married this hot young lawyer who was going to make lots of money and buy four dogs and live in a big house in Nashville's posh Belle Meade area and then . . .

She came home one night, extremely tired, and simply asked him to leave. She said she did not love him anymore and would he just go? That's Al's story, though I suspect there's more to it. Nevertheless, she left, and Al never got over the shock and hurt and resentment. It returned each time he had to find a ride to the hospital; each time he wanted to see his daughter, and couldn't, thinking it might be the last time; each time he thought about the man his wife was seeing.

The day I called his family's house, his father was out fishing, his mother was in South Carolina, and the help had the day off.

"Hey," I said. "How are you doing?"

"Fine," he said. "How are you doing?"

"How's your mom? And Heather? What's your dad been doing?"

"Come on, man. JUST TELL ME."

"Well, Al, looks like we might have a donor for you over in Knoxville. We're going over there in a little while and take a look. Why don't you take a shower, do whatever you need to do, and come on into the hospital. It'll be later tonight before we know for sure."

He couldn't reach his dad on the boat. He called South Carolina, but his aunt said his mom was out visiting friends. No one answered the phone at his old house, the one he once had lived in with his daughter and his wife. He took a taxi to the hospital.

When he woke up from surgery there was this huge face peering at him. Weird looking face. With little goggles or lights or something.

"Do you recognize me, Al? This is Dr. Frist."

200

"Where's my watch?" he said. He had always wanted a Rolex watch. Two or three weeks ago, he had said to himself, Well, I'm gonna die, and went out and bought the watch. He had been loath to give it up when he checked into the hospital. And now he wanted it back.

"Do you know who I am?" the strange face asked. It didn't seem to care about his watch.

"Yes," Al said. "You're Dr. Frist. You're very pretty, you know. Now, where's my damn watch?"

The surgery brought Suzanne and Al back together for a while. They tried, hard, to make a go of their marriage, but it was too late. They lasted only long enough to get rid of most of the bitterness between them. Not long after they split up the second time, Al discovered just how attractive a thirty-five-year-old hotshot good-looking lawyer could be. As his reputation with women spread through the office, all the doubts about him being some kind of invalid vanished. He became something of a folk hero in the Nashville legal community. A friend of his had even told him about a federal judge telling his favorite bartender about the near-dead lawyer who got a new heart and went wild.

Though his new lifestyle worried me, there was something about Al I could not help but approve of. He had thought long and deeply about life during the months when he thought he would die, and now he simply wanted to appreciate every single moment available to him. He would come into the office in his chic new casual clothes, wearing his Rolex watch, his thin dark moustache carefully trimmed, his eyes wrinkling like Clark Gable's, his whole being wrapped up in a dazzling smile that said, Ah, ain't life grand!

Al was the last patient I saw in clinic the day Jimmy Moore first broached the subject of a bicycle trip across the state. I had already checked over Ron Wynn, a middle-aged black patient who had had a transplant last year; he had added a large spare tire of fat around his middle. Ron had been a tough case, one who kept bleeding after transplantation, which forced me to operate again and again. By the time I finally pulled him out of it, his wife had heard me say, "I have to go back in, but there's nothing to worry about," so many times that I thought she was going to strike me with her fist. When I came in to tell her he was out of danger, before I could speak she yelled, "Don't you tell me you have to operate again! What's the matter with you, you can't get it right!"

Ron worked for DuPont, but the company's insurance did not cover his operation and his medicines. Several years back, when he first developed cardiomyopathy, he had been told then that someday he would have to have a transplant, but his heart mysteriously stopped deteriorating. He had just gone in for a regular checkup, the doctor had looked him over, and his heart was working normally. The doctor asked him if he had been praying, and Ron said he had, and the doctor ran around the hospital shouting that a miracle had occurred. It was a miracle that lasted five years. After his transplant, DuPont did not have a place for him at work but did continue his disability pay. Ron was doing great, enjoying life to the fullest, picking up odd jobs, participating in community activities.

I had also seen my star, the young deer hunter Mark Johnson, who was doing splendidly except for some aching joints from the steroids he was taking. I had reduced the dosage and sent him on his way. Back at work, with his family, no serious medical problems, exercising every day—Mark, too, was right on course.

Mark, like Ron before him, had asked me about Jimmy Moore's bike trip across the state. I had begun to suspect that Jan was secretly priming them when I walked in to check over Al Moore.

"So what's the verdict, Doc?" Al said.

"The verdict on what?" I asked, cautiously.

"On the bike trip, of course."

"I knew it," I said. "Jan put you up to this."

"No way," Al said. "We came up with this little baby on our own. Just think about it, Dr. Frist, how it would benefit all of us. Think of Ron. He needs the exercise if anybody ever did, and something to do. He's going crazy at home, even thinking about writing a book. And we certainly don't want that. It'll give Mark a chance to flex his muscles, Jimmy Moore an opportunity to stand up and blow off steam. And if I'm in training, I won't be out running around all night getting these dark circles under my eyes."

"Don't play lawyer with me," I laughed.

"Just one professional to another."

"I won't lie to you—"

"Dr. Frist, you can lie to me all you want. You do anyway, telling me how great things are, what a future I've got. And what gets me is I believe you. You could tell me this time you were going to chop off my head, sew it on another body, and that would be the best thing for me, and I'd say, 'Let's go, right now.' Just don't tell me you can't figure out some way that we can do this safely."

"I can't figure out—"

"Come on, man. Don't deny us this. Look, we're all grateful for what we've got. We want to give something back, let people know about the donor shortage, get people involved, make them aware. We want other people to have the opportunity that we have had. And who would be better spokespersons? Imagine it, front page, all of us standing with our bikes, big, healthy, handsome, Ron sucking in his gut of course."

I waved him quiet and somehow managed to finish the examination.

They were right. Ultimately, it was Billy Jones's miserable voice that convinced me: You got to have a donor to get one. I kept hearing it, and I kept thinking about all those people on my list.

Like Hugh Trigg, who would go on the list tonight. And like Billy Jones, who would not. Like Charles Stout up on Seven North, dying fast as he waited helplessly for a donor heart, who had said to me when I talked to him about his operation, "I don't want it. I'd rather die than saddle my family with the expense." Like Belinda Moreau, a beauty queen from Arkansas who had come to me because she couldn't raise the cash to get in at Texas. And like Jullie Haynes, also from Arkansas, waiting for a heart-lung operation. She also couldn't raise the cash.

Belinda and Jullie had met when their public fund-raising efforts in the same state had caused people to confuse them. Belinda had suggested they run a joint campaign. She had told Jullie about me and the Nashville program. And I had called Jullie and then, after evaluating her, put her on the list, too. Months later—long, hard, awful months—Belinda died waiting for a heart. The night before she asked to talk to me. She knew she was dying, and she said, "Please, I want the money I raised to go to Jullie. And I want her to get my donor. The heart you would have used for me." And Jullie was still waiting for that heart and lungs.

Today I had seen the lucky ones, the ones fortunate enough to receive donor hearts. The transplant didn't get rid of all of their problems, and indeed it introduced a number of problems they did not have before the procedure. But in the most fundamental way it gave their lives back to them, with all the glory and hell of any life. Jimmy Moore was macho before his transplant and macho after it. Hal Buckley drove himself too hard before and would probably drive himself too hard in the future. Ron Wynn, Mark Johnson, Al Moore were all essentially the same people, living in what were really only incidentally changed circumstances. They had the chance to fight their own particular demons. Dick Gibson did not, and neither did Belinda Moreau. Billy Jones wouldn't ever have that chance. Charles Stout, Hugh Trigg, and Jullie Haynes, one of them at least would probably not have it. If a bike trip got us even one more donor. . . .

I caught Jan as she was packing up to leave for dinner.

"Where's Jimmy Moore? Did he go back to South Carolina?"

"No," she said. "He's staying the night at the Med Center Inn. He leaves tomorrow."

"Jimmy?" I said when he answered the telephone.

"Dr. Frist?"

"OK. You can have your bike marathon. But we're going to do it my way."

Part Five

STARS

1

Jim Hayes inspired Jimmy Moore and company's trip across Tennessee, but it was one bike ride Jim Hayes could not make himself.

A month after his transplant, we managed to bring Jim out of his first episode of rejection. We discharged him across the street to the medical-center apartment house for patients and their families. Some who roomed there were on the waiting list, too sick to risk staying at home, but not so sick that they required hospitalization. Other tenants had a relative in critical care, someone who desperately needed a heart and who was fast running out of time. Still others, like Jim, were postoperative patients. I saw no reason to make them continue to pay the high costs of a hospital room, but we needed them close-by so we could see them in the clinic daily for a few weeks.

I especially wanted to keep an eye on Jim. He had developed a low-grade infection beneath the incision we had made on his chest. He then developed a bacterial pneumonia, associated with fever and malaise. We readmitted him. We cut back on his immunosuppression just a bit in order to treat his infections more aggressively. But with this he had another episode of rejection. This episode was severe enough to cause a fall in blood pressure, so we elected to treat the rejection with a powerful new drug called OKT3, a synthetic immunosuppressant and a monoclonal antibody, a drug we reserve for life-threatening episodes of rejection. Jim reacted violently to the drug, as patients occasionally do with the first dose. He became even more hypotensive, his falling blood pressure requiring treatment with pressor agents, including dopamine.

A new abnormality developed on his chest radiograph, the

diagnosis of which required an open-lung biopsy, a minor chest operation in a normal individual but more serious for Jim. The diagnosis of an aspergillus fungal infection was made. As we tried to treat both his infection and his rejection over the next few days, Jim's kidneys failed. By the middle of his second month post-op, he was back on the ventilator, requiring full lung-function support. That first night we intubated him, Shirley was standing outside Jim's CCU room, watching the machines breathe for her husband, when a young medical intern struck up a conversation with her. When he found out she was Jim's wife, he said, "That's Jim Hayes?"

"Yes," she said. "That's him."

"I—," said the intern, looking away.

"What?" Shirley asked. "What is it? Tell me!"

"I don't know how to—we were just talking about him."

"What is the matter?" Shirley almost screamed. "I have a right to know! I want to know."

The intern stared straight at her. "He's not going to make it. He's going to die. We think within twenty-four hours."

When I heard what had happened, I was furious, but I bit back on my anger. It would do no good now to chew out the inexperienced young intern. I had seen too much of that during my own residency. Instead, I thought, I needed to find Shirley as quickly as possible and undo as much of the psychological damage he had caused as I could. I caught up with her that afternoon in the visitors' waiting room. As I tried to talk to her she would not meet my eyes. She thought I had betrayed her.

"Shirley," I said, "I've always shot straight with you, always given you all of the information and told you what I was thinking, haven't I?"

She nodded.

"So listen when I tell you it's not over yet."

Her eyes flicked up, then away again.

"We have inexperienced people here. You know that. Remember all the trouble Jim had with his first biopsy last year? We have some people who don't know much about transplantation. People who haven't seen the ups and downs of the treatment before. I have. I won't lie to you. It does look bad. Jim is a very sick man. But it's not over yet. Trust me."

During the next two weeks, Jim improved, though very slowly. As the leaves on the trees turned colors outside his hospital room, the infection in his chest slowly cleared. At the end of his third month post-op, I let him go home for two weeks to be with Shirley and his son and to see his thirteen-year-old daughter by his first marriage, who was beginning to show disturbing signs of the anger that most neglected teenagers exhibit. The day Jim left, I found the young intern who had pronounced his imminent demise.

"We discharged Jim Hayes today. He went home to visit with his family," I said.

"That's great, Dr. Frist," he said nervously. "Just great."

"It wasn't twenty-four hours," I said. "And he's not dead."

Two weeks later Jim came back for another biopsy. The results showed that Jim's body was again attempting to attack his new heart. For the first time, I became afraid that Jim might be suffering from chronic, unrelenting rejection of his new heart. I tried to hide my discouragement from Shirley and from Jim, but I was frankly quite worried.

For more than eleven years, Jim Hayes had been a great example of the success of transplantation, celebrated not only within my narrow professional world but to an extent in the world at large. Years ago, millions had heard his story on "That's Incredible!" which had helped dispel the then-prevailing notion that heart-transplant patients were virtual invalids. The mayor of Knoxville had declared the day Jim left for his bike trip as Jim Hayes Day.

But now Jim was becoming an example of something else, of all that could go wrong with transplants. His first new heart had developed the accelerated atherosclerosis that some researchers speculated was a result of low-grade rejection. Not only had he suffered infections in his surgical incisions and lungs, but nagging lesions had appeared on his hands from longstanding cases of herpes. Now, he was having repeated biopsies—heart biopsies, lung biopsies, skin biopsies. And each infection we found only complicated the recurrent episodes of rejection striking him again and again with increasing frequency.

My treatment was already unconventional. At the time, OKT3 was used only for treating single episodes of severe rejection, for salvage therapy of life-threatening rejection. It was a new drug, very effective, but many feared a patient might develop antibodies to it if too much was used too soon; if so, the drug would be useless for fighting subsequent severe rejection episodes. They would treat such rejection once, and once only, with OKT3. By this time I had already tried steroids and RATG. Jim would not clear the rejection with these agents. He did respond to repeated treatments with OKT3, but once the drug was stopped, he would immediately start to reject again.

What else could I do? I couldn't operate again so soon, even if I found him another new heart, because his ongoing infections put him at too high a risk. The chances were that he would not survive the surgery; if he did, chances were that he would reject the next heart as well. I was being pushed to the very limits of my clinical knowledge of transplant immunology and biology. I felt forced into a corner, ordering dose after dose of OKT3 for Jim, a radical regimen that was only marginally successful, and a regimen that could not be continued indefinitely.

On dreary October nights, I found myself sitting at my desk flipping through stacks of phone messages, thinking about Jim Hayes. This field is just too young, I'd say to myself. We don't know enough. It's all word of mouth, or something picked up at a conference, maybe, or a clue hidden away in an inconclusive research report published in some obscure medical journal. There was no textbook to consult, no rules to follow.

The approach of the Thanksgiving holidays led both Shirley and Jim to ask when he would be discharged. I quickly put a stop to all such talk. I did not tell them my worst fears, but I did make it clear that while I might be able to move him into the hospital apartments before Thanksgiving, I nevertheless felt they should stay nearby for another month or two. As it turned out, Jim only lasted one day on the outside before he spiked a fever and, quite literally, began to lose his mind.

A virus had been attacking Jim's lungs. Now it infected his brain. We had no idea where the virus had come from, did not know its etiology. All we knew was that Jim had meningoencephalitis, and that ended any notion I had of retransplanting him. I had asked myself all along whether it would be right to give Jim yet another heart when so many people were waiting for their first transplant, dying for lack of a donor. But I had held the possibility in the back of my mind: if we got him well enough, if a heart became available, I might give it a try. But meningoencephalitis, like each of Jim's other infections, was an absolute contraindication to transplantation.

Jim's memory had gone by the time we had the neurosurgeons place an Ommaya reservoir inside his skull to decompress the swollen brain ventricles and relieve the pressure that was squashing his brain against his skull. Day by day, his blood pressure fell, he went into shock, and he just got sicker and sicker. I had to support his heart with powerful drugs just so his blood would circulate and keep his brain, his kidneys, and his liver alive. He barely responded to the drugs, and we reintubated him, put him once again back on the ventilator.

In late November, Jim Hayes sank into a deep coma. It was painful just making rounds on him in the ICU everyday, seeing him lying in such a miserable state, so lifeless and unresponsive.

Now I had more than some green intern to contend with. At a Christmas party, one of the hospital's cardiologists, a highly respected medical doctor, approached Karyn and casually mentioned that I was really going overboard with Jim Hayes. He suggested I was too personally and emotionally involved in the case, told her that my unrelenting efforts bordered on an obsession that kept me from seeing the truth: Jim Hayes could not possibly survive. The consensus around Vanderbilt, he said, was that I should simply let the poor man die. Karyn conveyed the message, of course, as I am sure he had intended she should. I realized that the time might be coming when I would have to face such charges from my superiors.

That night the trauma unit received a gunshot victim, and I had to return to the hospital. On the way back in, I found myself wondering if the cardiologist was right. Jim Hayes had exhausted all currently available medicines for treating rejection. I had already run risks most others would not have run, or at least had not yet run.

The man I operated on that night was about Jim's size and age. One bullet had hit his heart directly, leaving a hole big enough to put my fist into, and the procedure was dramatic and bloody and exhausting. The surgery lasted some five hours. At one point I thought we would pull the fellow through, despite the extensive damage to his heart and the massive loss of blood. Then his body gave a little flop. The heart had arrested. We shocked it back to life, and for nearly forty-five minutes I massaged it, my hands buried deep in his chest till they grew cramped and stiff. I stepped side and allowed my surgical assistant to massage for a few minutes, then started up again when I could flex my fingers.

In the end, the patient died. He had suffered not only the heart wound but also severe damage to several other organs from a second bullet and from massive intra-abdominal bleeding. By the time I decided to call a halt to the operation, I could see the fatigue in the sloped shoulders and vacant stares of the others in the room. We shut off the ventilator.

It happens. Just let the poor man die, I thought, as I headed for my office, drained and a bit depressed. When I got there, I flicked through the telephone messages on my desk, saw nothing that needed attention that late at night, and flipped on the computer. I called up Jim's file. The screen blinked, there was a little beep, and up came the words "Formatted Total Data Listing." I scrolled down from "Hayes, Jim. Demographic #141 Registry TX-19" to item number ninety-six. It read:

96- Comment on clinical course to date:

18 JUN : Hypotensive postop; extubated on 4th POD.
23 JUN : Dopamine, PA line; Rejection, severe. Sick.
30 JUN : Jim has hand lesion which has been scraped for diagnosis of herpes in the past. This recurs and acyclovir is started with good resolution.
3 JUL : Rejection # 2.

10 JUL : Discharged to apartment.

23 JUL : Rehospitalized for mediastinitis (staph coagulase negative)

3 AUG : Lung failure. On ventilator. Renal failure. Violent reaction OKT3. Renal failure. Rejecting heart.

11 SEP : Rehospitalized for treatment of refractory rejection with OKT3.

24 SEP : Recurrent severe rejection.

7 OCT : Readmitted to treat rejection. Episode # 6.

12 OCT : Patient was treated with amphotericin from 10/20 to 11/7. Biopsy of lung mass on 10/17 revealed staph aureus, and aspergillus. Absolute contraindication to retransplant.

18 NOV : Discharged yesterday. Now has fever. Loss of memory. Readmit today.

25 NOV : Comatose. Reintubated. Prognosis dismal.

1 DEC : Ommaya reservoir placed to decompress ventricles of brain. Brain biopsy #1: Negative.

10 DEC : Brain biopsy #2: Negative, comatose. Magnetic resonance imaging shows multiple brain masses.

"Twenty Dee Eee Cee colon," I said aloud. "Simply let the poor man die." I rubbed my eyes. It's late, I thought. One of those nights. I've been here before. I felt the way I had as an intern up in Boston when that young girl, the burn victim, had died on my watch. I waited too long then, I thought, to call for help. I did not believe Ed Stinson would have any answers for me as I reached for the telephone and dialed his home number in California, but it was two in the morning and I needed to talk to somebody who would at least understand what I was going through. Precisely what I was going through.

It was midnight his time, but he was a transplant surgeon and scientist, and he would find what I had to say fascinating.

"Ed, this is Bill. Bill Frist."

"Bill?" There was a pause. I imagined him reaching for a lamp by the bed. Holding up an alarm clock. Knitted brows. "Good to hear from you. Where are you?"

"Here," I said. "Here in Nashville. I know you think I'm crazy

213

for calling so late, but I'm a little bit lonely here, and I really need to bounce some ideas off you."

"So what have you got going on?" Ed said in his customary matter-of-fact way. How I missed that dry, no-nonsense tone, so clinical, so smart, so ultimately humane if you knew where to look for the hidden passion.

"Remember Walter Packman?" I said, gearing up to talk about Jim. Ed had a real affection for my patient, having been in charge of the Stanford program when Jim had his first operation. "The eleven-year-old boy with recurrent rejection? The one we gave two hundred rads of total lymphoid radiation?"

"Yes," Ed said.

"It seemed to cure him."

"Yes."

Total lymphoid radiation was very unconventional therapy for the treatment of rejection. Years ago Stanford had been involved in early studies of the radiation therapy, but had never clearly demonstrated its clinical usefulness. Now that we had other, more specific immunosuppressant agents, nobody bothered much with radiation. Still, in usual Stanford style, Stinson had kept an open mind, using the therapy as a last resort on the young Packman child. It seemed to work, though there was no scientific evidence, no clinical proof, that it would and no prospective clinical trial to demonstrate its efficacy. But when you are working in a new field, one full of unknowns and the unexpected, you don't always have the luxury of having well-accepted recipes to choose from. Just my asking would cue Ed that I faced something serious.

"Bill, is this about Walter Packman?" he asked.

"No," I said. "It's about Jim Hayes."

I told him everything that had happened, including the comment from the cardiologist earlier that night. I knew that Stinson had always been a proponent of retransplantation. He had insisted that anybody who engaged seriously in heart transplants must be prepared to embark on retransplantation if the need arose. It was an obligation of sorts. After a patient's fourth episode

214

of rejection, Stinson had always said one should move directly to retransplantation.

"Ed," I said, "would it be advisable to give Jim Hayes yet a third transplant? You always said after twelve rounds of Solu-Medrol, you've gotta do it. He's had his twelve rounds. Right now, Jim's comatose and has meningoencephalitis."

"You've tried all other therapies," he said, more as a fact than a question.

"That's right. The usual steroid regimen. I've tried everything. I've even given him Cytoxan." Cytoxan was a drug commonly used to treat cancer. "And I've used OKT3 repeatedly. Six times in a row."

"You've used OKT3 serially *six times?*" Stinson said, stunned, perhaps even dismayed. "We've started using it prophylactically right after surgery. For a single episode of severe refractory rejection later. We've never used it serially in the same patient. The drug company has not approved it for that."

"It's the only therapy he's responding to," I said.

"You've used OKT3 six times, and he's responding to it? Amazing." Ed was hooked now. I could almost hear the wheels turning in his head through the fiberoptics of the long-distance network. "Bill," he said. "I know you've thought about all this, but it seems to me you have three alternatives. You can retransplant Jim. That's your decision to make, nobody else's, and don't let the talk get you down. But it's a tough one, with this ongoing infection of his. You are probably looking at a sixty percent chance of mortality. And you've got others on your list whose chances are much better.

"You can do what you're doing. Keep using OKT3 as you are. But, as you know, Jim will never leave the hospital; he'll always have some sort of infection as long as you keep it up. On the other hand, you say he's responding right now, and maybe some better drug will come along.

"The third alternative, as I see it, is the one you really called about. You can go ahead with the radiation. We have not radiated any one here since Walter Packman, and you know how that

215

went. We have nothing to say it will work with Jim, nothing definitive, but it seemed to work that one time. It's only anecdotal. Maybe we should give it another try?"

The "we" in his sentence heartened me in a way I hadn't experienced for a long time. It was another thing I loved about the specialty of transplantation, the sense that we were all in this together, learning from one another as the new field grew, evolved, changed. There were controversies, and the debates could be heated, but as soon as anyone uncovered something new, he immediately passed it along to his colleagues around the country.

"Is anybody else using lymphoid irradiation?" I asked.

"Not to my knowledge," Ed said. "You might give some of those who participated in the initial study a call. When I get to the office tomorrow I'll find the names and numbers for you."

"What dosages of radiation should I use?"

"I think it's fairly arbitrary," he said. "Talk to your radiation therapist at Vanderbilt, but I'd start treatment immediately giving one hundred rads five days a week till we see a response."

"I'm going to do it," I said. There was an awkward pause. "This is what I miss most about Stanford," I said. "You always told me there were no clear-cut answers to any of this, and I understand that, but I miss bouncing ideas off of everyone."

"Let's hope it's a good idea we're bouncing off here," Ed said. "Let me know what happens."

As soon as I put the phone down, I started to plan how tomorrow I'd call the others and talk to Vanderbilt's radiation therapist. With some pleasure, I imagined the surprise on his face when I outlined "our" unconventional approach. Then, with a start, I realized I hadn't even wished Ed a Merry Christmas.

I had on my bookshelf a row of videocassettes, and as the night crept toward dawn I pulled out two of them. One was a short ten-minute tape of a rare public appearance by both Shumway and Stinson at a national transplant meeting. Impossible, I thought. That never happened. The two of them together. On the same podium. But there it was. The other was the segment from the old "That's Incredible!" program covering Jim Hayes's bike trip to Stanford.

I went into the office kitchen down the hall and made myself a pot of coffee. Steaming cup in hand, I found the VCR in the copy room and popped in the Shumway-Stinson tape.

Shumway, at the podium, looked relaxed, laid-back, a devilish grin stretched across his face as he gave a hilarious rendition of the history of heart transplants. It was a shame Shumway did not speak more often, because he was so good at it.

"There are seven stages," he said "that happen in the development of any new idea, and these apply particularly to surgery. In the first stage, doubters all around you say, 'It won't work; it's never been tried before.' After several successful experiences with animals, you enter the second stage, and the same doubters say, 'But it won't work in man.' One successful clinical patient later, they turn around, shake their heads, and mumble, 'Very lucky. But the patient really did not need the operation in the first place. Too bad the tragedy occurred; they'll probably try it again.'"

Instead of simply letting the poor man die, I thought.

"After four or five clinical experiences, critics call it 'highly experimental. Too risky. Probably immoral. Certainly unethical.' And someone in the back adds in a whisper, 'I understand that they probably had a number of deaths that they have not reported.' The fifth stage is characterized by critics saying, after ten or fifteen successful patients, 'May proceed cautiously in carefully selected cases, but most patients with this defect don't need the operation anyway.' In the sixth stage, after a large series of successes, some critics say, 'I hear that a number of their patients are now dying late deaths,' while other critics are saying, 'So-and-so elsewhere cannot get the same results.' Finally, in the seventh stage, the critics now say, 'I know this is a very fine contribution. A straightforward solution to a difficult problem. I predicted this. In fact, I had the same idea long before they even started. Of course, we didn't publish.'"

I was waiting for it, that sly smile, and then: "These are a few of the comments that I have heard over the last twenty-five years in our work in heart transplantation."

By contrast, Ed Stinson appeared even more awkward than normal when he walked into view and eyed the mike as if it were some kind of snake trying to hypnotize him. His dry, toneless voice recounted the clinical history of the field. By the time he should have been finished, he was still talking about the 101 procedures done at two dozen centers around the world in the twelve months after Chris Barnard—both Shumway and Stinson always called him Chris, as if he were their little brother—had become the new Dr. Frankenstein.

But it was only Ed's tone that was dry. "I would say to you without any hint of arrogance or overconfidence that Stanford's perseverance through this time—through these doldrums of heart transplantation during the 1970s—served an important contribution in preserving not only scientific, but also societal interest in clinical cardiac transplantation. We were like babies crying in the wilderness—shouting in the wilderness would be a more apt expression. The message that we were attempting to deliver was that clinical heart transplantation constitutes a viable therapeutic procedure."

"Amen," I said. And, lifting my Styrofoam coffee cup, "Merry Christmas, Ed." The South African, good old Chris Barnard, had once compared a transplant patient to a man standing on the edge of a river filled with crocodiles, with a lion rushing at him. He either got eaten by the lion or he made a leap of faith to swim to the other side. Jim had made that leap, and I was supposed to be there to help him across. I plunged the next tape into the VCR.

The female host of "That's Incredible!" came on, introducing Jim through a series of takes that showed him in physical therapy, looking muscled and healthy, his surgical scar quite invisible among the hair on his chest. He looked thirty years younger than he did now, not merely eight or so. Suddenly there he was in Knoxville with his skinny brother, their bikes loaded up, the mayor leading the crowd to see them off. When they tracked his six-week cross-country route on a map, it reminded me of the

218

beginning of *Casablanca*. They interrupted the graphics with interviews of Jim at stops along the way. There he was complaining about the headwinds in Kansas. Next, he was standing atop the Rockies, snow swirling around him, talking through his nose about the cold he had picked up.

Good lord, I had forgotten that. He had actually caught a cold! Then there was a shot of the Palo Alto exit sign off the interstate that made me even more nostalgic. And a picture of Jim and his brother roaring up into a cheering crowd standing in front of the hospital. And shots of his yearly checkup. And a special sort of shot, I don't know what you'd call it, kind of like a bulletin board with three or four postcards stuck on it, each showing different moving images from the segment, as circus-poster letters typed themselves magically over the screen: "Incredible Courage!"

The milky sun, a pale ghost of itself, hung in the early morning mist as I made my way across the street to my frost-encrusted car. I suppose I had intended to head home, but I found myself turning the wrong way, driving down the ramp onto I-40, motoring past Metro Airport and pulling up in front of the private strip where my old Apache had sat waiting patiently for me throughout most of a year.

An hour later I was airborne, looping my way around Nashville in a cold, midwinter sky.

2

The things she had seen. Holley Cully told herself she shouldn't get hooked, but she could not help it. There was Jimmy Moore, sicker than a dog, highly infectious, and she just shouldn't get attached. Then going down there to cardiac recovery. And they'd say he was doing fine, but he wouldn't open his eyes. Standing outside the room, her nose pressed against the glass, for days. Then one morning there was a flicker of eyelids, and before she could get her mask on he gave her the thumbs-up sign.

And good old happy-go-lucky Ron Wynn, smiling like a sunny day and riding the stationary bike in his room to beat the devil and then—she was working evenings and came out of report and walked into his room—he was lying across the bed and he had absolutely no blood pressure. Well, like 40 systolic, and she got things going and got the doctors up there and, well, he was cardiac tamponading from all the blood accumulating around his heart. The first time she had ever seen it. You know, she'd heard about it, but you don't ever see it. Hardly. Well, Ron did that twice on her in recovery and once down in the unit. Down in the unit these transplant patients had a bad habit of doing bad things like that when she was on duty, but, Lord, she was hooked.

Jim Hayes was the worst. The New Year was still a babe in arms and she had taken care of that man for six months. When you see something like that, someone like Jim—was this his twelfth year? She knew she was looking at a miracle, because he was the biggest fighter, because he had beaten the odds more than anybody, but he'd come back in with horrible, horrible infections, and now the coma. She'd think, Well, is this transplantation really the thing, you know? She'd find herself lying in bed, the baby finally asleep, and she'd think, He just can't take any more. She'd pray to God, Just let him go, just let him go.

"Then Dr. Frist," Holley would tell it, "Dr. Frist, it was incredible—Jim was so sick, you know, and I was almost afraid to ask Dr. Frist what he was doing to Jim, now. It was all so weird with radiation like Jim had cancer, but Dr. Frist was the eternal optimist and he'd shoot straight with you, too, and he'd walk up—he'd kind of blast through the floor and you'd have to catch him on the run—and he'd stop me sometimes and say, 'Holley, I'm gonna pull him through this for you. I swear, I'm going to pull him through.' And Shirley, she would come up and tell me over and over again, 'He's gonna be back.'

"So, sure, when I heard them talking on the floor about removing all of Jim's life support, I would think, Yes, yes. Let's end this and at the same time be thinking that Jim Hayes did not want to give up and so, by God, I wouldn't. They had moved him up to the floor, about as close to dead as he could get, tubes out of every orifice he had, though they said there were signs that he was improving, maybe coming out of his coma. Yeah. Right. Dr. Frist, Chief of Optimism at Vanderbilt University Medical Center, talking.

"Then that little turkey, he woke up. Scared me to death. I couldn't believe it. Two days later I walked in the room and—from nowhere—Jim Hayes had said, 'Hi, Holley, how you doing?' Well I just lost it, you know? My face was just down on his chest and I was just bawling my eyes out, and Jim, he was patting me, and saying, 'That's all right. That's all right.' And I sat down on the floor and cried."

The things she'd seen.

Formatted Total Data Listing

Hayes, Jim. Demographic #141 Registry TX-19

96- Comment on clinical course to date:

221

27 JAN : Extubated. Jim began to wake up three days ago. Has been maintained on the ventilator for the past 64 days.

14 FEB : Out of bed, walking. Still has poor memory, but looks great.

17 MAR : Clinically doing well. Asymptomatic.

25 MAR : Reinitiation of radiation therapy today with plans to deliver a total of 1500 rads.

31 MAR : Has received 240 rads of total lymphoid irradiation at Vanderbilt.

12 MAY : Memory improving daily. Saw eye doctor: no change in prescriptions. Reading well.

19 MAY : No problems except urinary frequency.

26 MAY : Exercising 3× week; TLI 2× week.

By early summer, Jim Hayes was attending clinic regularly, coming down from his hospital room under his own power with Shirley, and piecing his life back together. His memory still failed him often, but occasionally he would come out with a direct comment or statement that made you realize the Jim Hayes of "That's Incredible!" was yet inside him, struggling mightily to spring forth and face the world. On one of those visits, Jim shook his head as if he were a heavyweight fighter shrugging off a good blow during a mandatory eight count. He said, "Hey, Doc, what's this I hear about a bike trip?"

"Don't even think about it, Jim," I said.

But he wanted to know, so I told him. I told him Jimmy Moore had taken his inspiration from Jim's trip to Stanford and that we had been planning the trip for nearly a year. I told him that we had found a corporate sponsor to underwrite the costs, an employee-benefits company called Equicor. Murray Ohio Manufacturing Company was supplying custom-made touring bikes. I told him that Jay Groves had the whole gang—Jimmy, Mark Johnson, Al Moore, and Ron Wynn—down in his exercise room three times a week working on their endurance.

"You remember, Jim," Shirley coaxed. "We saw them down there."

222

"We did?"

"Uh-huh. That's when Jimmy told you about it."

"That's right," Jim said. "Ron Wynn is going, too?"

"He sure is. If he can get himself in shape in time," I said.

We started holding meetings almost every week to discuss the trip. Equicor was represented by the president of a local public-relations firm the company hired. Sometimes he would bring his media experts, who had the thankless task of trying to teach the others around the table how to deal with television coverage. The others consisted of the likes of Jay Groves and Jan Muirhead, Walter Merrill, Dr. Bob Richie, who was in charge of the kidney-transplant program at Vanderbilt, and several organ-donor coordinators and their bosses from the regional organ-procurement agencies in the Southeast.

Equicor was quite a coup for us. The company had taken the lead in the insurance field by covering all transplant operations, including heart-lungs, for those who worked in the organizations it insured. They covered the increased costs by deducting a few extra cents each month from all of the company's employees. Equicor was a savvy organization. It realized that heart-transplant therapy, far from being still in the experimental phase, was now being looked at as a model for the practice of all other types of high-tech medicine.

In 1986 Medicare, the huge federal program that provides health-insurance coverage for the elderly, extended coverage to its beneficiaries for heart transplants. Medicare would pay only those transplant programs that met stringent survival and experience criteria set by the Health Care Financing Administration. Because the HCFA required a program to be three years old and to have performed at least twelve operations each year, the new rules were especially hard on young programs like ours.

But more importantly, for the first time in the history of health-care legislation the government focused on the quality of the therapy it would reimburse. A decade ago, the government had argued that the primary criterion for acceptable medical care should be its accessibility to all those in need. In the mid-1970s,

Congress passed legislation aimed at making dialysis and kidney transplants available to all, regardless of success rates. Now, in contrast, heart transplant centers were required not just to perform a given number of operations but to achieve success rates that matched those at Stanford and the other leading programs. It was the wave of the future.

Insurance companies like Equicor would play a dominant role in that future. Perhaps more than for any other procedure, private and public insurance for heart transplantation has been varied. The expenses for heart transplantation were beyond the private means of all but the very wealthy. We simply had to develop some form of third-party payment to cover our increasingly expensive medical care. Insurance coverage for heart transplants has been added by most major insurers to the package of benefits available for employers to select. Basic benefit packages that include transplantation must be encouraged, if not mandated, either by public pressure or possibly more appropriately by state governments, which are responsible for regulating the conditions under which private health insurance coverage is offered in each state.

The best bet was still private insurance, but it was hit or miss. What got paid for depended on how well you were covered. But some thirty-seven million Americans had absolutely no medical coverage for any type of illness. Even if a patient managed to pay for the transplant operation, the costs continued. Medical bills became a devastating part of life for many, even a defeat of life. After all, what was the point of having life-extending technology if the life it extended wasn't worth living? Why save someone's life physically, while wrecking it economically and psychologically? I could see the day coming when there would be no medical reason for any of us to die, but no way to finance the continued life we could provide. In 1988, medical expenses were eleven percent of the GNP, more than $540 billion. But as much as twenty-five percent of those health care costs were for things that were wasted or unnecessary. We simply had to develop some better system of third-party payment that would make access to health care more equitable, eliminate waste, and cover the escalating costs.

Equicor was justly proud of its leadership role. They saw Jimmy Moore's Famous Bike Trip, as I had dubbed it, as a way of trumpeting that pride. The company billed the event as the Equicor Organ Transplant Bikers Across Tennessee. But as they made plans to promote the trip—creating a logo, producing T-shirts, plastering signs on each of the growing number of vehicles that would accompany our bikers—they began to tread on the sensitive toes of our health-care professionals.

The organ-donor coordinators in the Vanderbilt conference room questioned Equicor's self-promotion and argued that we were losing our focus on the real purpose of the bike trip: donor awareness. The coordinators cared deeply about people, about helping potential transplants, about persuading more of the public to sign donor cards and donate organs.

But their arguments also had an economic edge. For a number of years following the widespread introduction of cyclosporine, heart-transplant operations had increased dramatically. Last year the rate at which they increased began to level off, and now it might even be dropping. The reason? The shortage of donors. As the number of heart transplants had increased, so had the number of transplant programs and the organ-procurement agencies who served them. The agencies were highly competitive; the HCFA had begun certifying agencies in an effort to eliminate some of that competition. Some organizations refused even to talk to us, while others jealously guarded their own regions, insisting on handling local arrangements themselves.

And, finally, there were the Vanderbilt people, trained doctors and nurses. They were uncomfortable with PR types, whom they didn't understand. And they were uncomfortable with the organ coordinators, whom they understood all too well, being both dependent on them and somewhat condescending about their "market orientation." They wanted to concentrate entirely on the patients making the trip, to ensure that they were healthy and safe.

Everybody was polite enough, but they were always talking at cross-purposes. I used to smile to myself thinking I ought to invite Jimmy Moore in to see how very complicated his simple idea had become. But he would only shake his head in bewilderment and say, "It's just us and a few bikes. We meet people all over the state, and we tell them to sit down and think about donating organs when they die. What's the problem?" As the discussions about portable telephones (to call the media, to call the local organizer, to call for emergency medicines) and cars (to show logos, to haul extra bikes, to store emergency medical equipment) ran on and on, I would think gleefully to myself, It's this whole complex field of transplantation in microcosm right before my eyes.

Transplantation involved a complicated notion of medical care, a new notion. It was unfamiliar and threatening beyond the Frankensteinish fears of the early days when state governments and city attorneys used to indict surgeons and charge them with murder for removing hearts from brain-dead patients. And because transplantation was a new and unique kind of treatment, it called upon the transplant surgeon to take steps outside the traditional surgeon's role. The transplant surgeon did things that other surgeons found odd. One of them was mediating competing interests like those in the conference room. Another was traveling about the country giving what I called my little talks.

Sometimes I would drive fifty miles, sometimes fly hundreds of miles. I went mostly to small community hospitals, but I also spoke to schools and civic groups and women's clubs. I came occasionally for lunch, often for dinner, and always for a talk afterward. I tried to squeeze as many of these meetings into my schedule as I could during my first two years at Vanderbilt because I knew the kind of mixed reactions, from awe to anger, that people had to our transplant efforts. And while I would much rather have spent my time with patients, I felt that no one could present the case of donor need to other physicians as well as one of their own. And it did not hurt for potential donors to hear a surgeon talk about the organ shortage. I was the one who watched waiting people die; I felt an obligation to speak for this group. Since closing the gap between available organs and dying recipients was essential if transplantation was to reach its lifesaving potential, I told myself I had no choice but to be a major part of the education process.

The talk varied a bit given the nature of the audience. Sometimes I'd show a videotape of the transplant operation itself, other times not, but my main points were always the same.

I gave a brief history of transplantation, including a slide of my mentor Norman Shumway, whom I proudly proclaimed the father of heart transplantation. I also usually included the legal and political history of the field, which was especially important to the physicians.

I told them about the development of the criteria for brain death as a legal definition of death and how the doctors who take out the organs cannot be the ones who pronounce the donor dead. I mentioned the Uniform Anatomical Gift Act, passed in 1968, which established the legal status of donor cards and living wills, as well as the right of the next of kin to make donations for relatives who had never indicated their opposition to serving as a donor. It created what we called encouraged voluntarism. This method of procuring organs had failed miserably, as the donor shortage indicated.

I talked about Senator Albert Gore's efforts to keep the system of procuring organs from being manipulated by appeals from prominent patients or a misguided president. Such manipulation had compromised the system in the past. Some donors had specified who got their organs. Wealthy foreigners who had donated large sums of money to medical centers had received organs before Americans. Senator Gore's efforts to prevent "list-jumping" led to the National Organ Transplant Act of 1984, which set up the nationwide system for matching donors and recipients, established a national task force on transplantation, authorized federal assistance for qualified organ-procurement agencies, and provided funding for the creation of a single, cohesive, twenty-four hour computerized network to handle all available donor organs.

I mentioned UNOS, the United Network for Organ Sharing

in Richmond, VA. This private organization had been awarded the federal contract in 1986 to ensure fair access to and allocation of donated organs. I tried to talk a little about the allotment system itself, which was still in flux, but which took into consideration distance, tissue and blood-type match, body size, degree of illness, and dependance on artificial life-supports. UNOS tried first to use an organ locally. If no suitable patient could be found, the organ was made available regionally, then nationally, all in a matter of minutes via computer.

And I pointed out that a recent federal law required hospitals to approach relatives of brain-dead patients about organ donation.

I always discussed the goals of transplantation, the quality of life issues. The goal was to return a terminally ill patient, someone who would otherwise die, to a functional lifestyle, a life as normal as possible given the side effects of immunosuppressant drugs and the risks of infection and rejection, all of which I described briefly. But I always stressed that the therapy was viable and effective, that patients lived full and productive lives. I showed slides of my youngest patient, Jonathan Jones, and my oldest, a sixty-three-year-old man from Stanford. Here, too, I would mention costs, pointing out that heart transplants were expensive, but that those costs were coming down rapidly as more experience was gained. Kidney transplants had once been expensive, too, even more expensive than hearts, but today they were generally accepted to be one of the most cost-effective therapies we had, freeing recipients from the astronomical price of dialysis.

I also drove home the team approach of transplantation and showed a slide with the patient and family at the center of a circle made up of the transplant surgeon, the referring physician, social workers, psychologists, nurses, physical therapists, financial counselors, pathologists, and community support groups. I made the point that the cure wasn't the surgery, but the overall commitment to the continued care of these recipients. Sometimes I would turn to the future, showing the LVAD and explaining its uses, describing how we were trying to increase the specificity of immunosuppression and look for a less invasive alternative to the frequent heart biopsies. I also suggested to the audience that they consider the benefits of a presumed-consent law that might allevi-ate some of the donor shortage.

I always ended with the donor shortage, hitting that point hardest of all. I showed a slide of a pie with 25,000 potential donors and our inexcusably small slice of only some 4,000 actual donors each year, of which only 1,700 were heart donors. And I pointed out that there were at least three times that many people who could benefit from heart transplantation on the basis of traditionally accepted criteria, adding that the indications and age limits for heart transplantation have continued to expand. At any point in time, there were over a thousand people on the UNOS computer list waiting for hearts. And there are many more who, for a multitude of reasons, never make it to these formal lists. As many as one out of four will die waiting.

And not only hearts: more than 16,000 people were on the official UNOS list for all organs. Thousands more—perhaps 100,000 people on any given day—needed new organs. The of-ficial waiting list reflected only those who had been lucky enough to make it into the medical-care system and to pass the financial hurdles. If you included all those coming to end-stage disease, the number waiting for organs became staggering. Only a fraction of that number would ever receive transplants—even if they had adequate insurance and enough money. Any one of us could need a transplant tomorrow, and the chances are we wouldn't get it, because there are not enough donors.

I talked about donor cards, how important they were not so much as legal documents, but as indications of a willingness to donate. We always asked the next of kin, regardless, and a donor card simply helped the loved ones make their choice. I urged members of the audience to use the signing of such a card as an opportunity to talk about organ donation with those closest to them, well in advance of the time when they might have to make hard decisions. And finally I gave the telephone number for UNOS, a number they could call twenty-four hours a day to ask any question whatsoever about organ donation: 1-800-24-DONOR.

Then I stepped back and waited for the questions. Sometimes, with the women's clubs and high-school groups, they were fairly benign; requests for information, calls for suggestions about how one individual could help. And others in the room, even doctors, would occasionally seem awestruck. I heard one young doctor remark to another at one of the rural hospitals, "This is it, the highest pinnacle of medicine. Those guys are the cream of the crop." But more often I thought that it was obvious that the physicians in the audience felt resentment, maybe jealousy at the field's high visibility. Sometimes anger seemed to crackle through the room on the back of their questions.

I remembered one in particular because he reminded me of the country doctor my father might have been had he stayed in Mississippi. Corduroy jacket, rumpled shirt, baggy pants, thick glasses, hair slicked back, he shifted uneasily in his seat, obviously disturbed, as I fielded the first question from a matronly nurse.

"Who can donate? I mean, are there limits?"

"We don't take anybody with a systemic disease, like cancer, or anyone who has an active infection. For hearts we generally don't like to take anyone over fifty because of the propensity to develop atherosclerosis. But otherwise anybody can donate tissues and organs. Anyone from infancy to seventy years old."

The old doc couldn't sit still any longer.

"I don't know about this forcing me to ask for organs such as the heart. I've already got Medicare and Medicaid telling me how much I get reimbursed for what I do, and I can tell you they are squeezing me dry. I've got HMOs who decide who I can admit and who I can't. Enough's enough."

I replied, "Well, what we have discovered is that someone has got to bring the subject up, to give a family the opportunity to donate. Many people find the subject of donation so tough to think about that they ignore general appeals, even when the polls consistently show that most of them are willing to dona—"

"You miss my point, doctor. I don't like the government telling me how to practice medicine. It is none of their business how I interact with my patients. I mean, I know these people, I've known them all my life. Been their doctor for twenty years. Their son dies, I'd feel like a vulture, some kind of ghoul asking to mutilate his body. I'm a physician, they expect me to console them at a time like that. Not badger them."

"Exactly. You're a physician, licensed by the state, certified by a legal medical board, and charged with a certain responsibility to the welfare of society. That includes your patients' feelings, but it also includes the health and life of the fifteen people who could use that son's tissues and organs. We, as physicians, are ghouls indeed if we don't let that family know it has an opportunity at that point in time—"

"It's just not American," he said. "These things must cost an arm and a leg."

"That's a problem. They are enormously expensive for the patient. A heart transplant costs as much as $100,000 the first year and then $6,000 to $10,000 in medicines and continued care every year after that. Almost all places require much of that fee up front. Very few people can pay that kind of money out of their own pockets. Government, Medicare, and third-party payers have slowly but steadily increased their reimbursements for the procedures, but many people are still denied transplants solely because they can't pay. On the other hand, historically, our society has been reluctant to withhold lifesaving medical treatments because of an inability to pay."

"You're talking socialized medicine. I mean, I sit here, and I listen to you, and I can't believe you are Dr. Tommy Frist's son. You let people die, for God's sake, because they don't fit on some computer. How can you play God like that?"

"That's why I need you to help me find more donors. So no one is asked to make those types of decisions. No one has to play God."

3

Very occasionally, my father would join me when I traveled to one of the small hospitals owned by HCA. He would use the occasion to visit with those he thought of as his people and to tour the facilities. I remembered one night in particular, in the small plane coming back from a meeting in west Tennessee, when the questions had been particularly pointed and the discomfort with transplantation and all it portended had been all but palpable in the hospital's stuffy little meeting room. A huge orange summer moon was clearing the horizon, and the series of little towns glowed in the dusty slow curve of the land below like a sunset gone flat.

I could see Dad was worried by the way he kept bobbing his head, not muttering aloud to himself, exactly, but doing whatever the mental equivalent of that might be. We had the lights turned down in the cabin, the better to watch the otherworldly beauty of the night, but I could still see his shadowy face in the light of the moon and the on-again-off-again red blink of our running lights. Now and then his eyes would flick over my face, quick, concerned, and when I caught him, he'd mouth "beautiful, just beautiful" against the loud drone of the engine and point with a long, graceful index finger toward the big round orb on the horizon.

The taciturn pilot, a man in his early fifties with a stiff military bearing and close-shaved white hair, often flew the planes I rented. I had learned to respect his skills, but had also come to realize that he did not feel comfortable with me sitting in the copilot's seat. So except during takeoffs and landings, when I simply couldn't help myself, these days and nights I mostly sat in the cabin when I had fellow passengers.

I had my back to the pilot, watching my dad, and I got up and moved over next to him and put my arm on his shoulder.

"What's troubling you?"

"That," Dad said, motioning with his head back toward the hospital. "Back there."

"Don't worry," I said cheerfully. "I'm used to it."

"Reminds me of when we were first starting out with HCA, and people hated the idea of investor-owned corporations running hospitals. Tommy and I would fly into these small towns and our reception would often be hostile. But with time, the reception warmed. Same kind of thing. Future blind."

We sat silently for a while, and I watched the thousands of little lights below turn to hundreds as we passed beyond the towns and out over the country and woods of middle Tennessee.

"Bill," Dad said, "I don't want to preach, but you ought to spend more time with your family. You are wearing yourself out with this. I know you feel strongly about your mission and all that, but you personally cannot reach everybody fast enough. You'll always be playing catch-up ball anyway."

"I know," I said. He was absolutely right. As I looked out at the lights below, dwindling now to dozens instead of hundreds, I could see that there was no connection between them, no common forum or meeting hall where I could say to enough of them, "We have people dying and we want you to help." There was nothing bringing them together but the electrical current that fed the lights and the abstract geography of the nation-state. Which left two ways of reaching them effectively: television and federal legislation.

If traveling around like some kind of evangelical minister, speaking to small groups of anybody who would listen, was strange behavior for a surgeon, appearing on network television with a country-music star was unheard of. I think even Barbara Mandrell herself was surprised at my naive willingness to go on the road with her, promoting transplant issues and a celebrity softball game for transplantation. She was totally dedicated to the cause, I discovered.

She turned out to be deeply religious in a freewheeling way. She had almost lost her life in 1984 in an automobile wreck, saved only by her fastened seat belt. She seemed enamored of the notion that one could make tragic death a life-giving proposition.

Barbara had bright, clear, intelligent blue eyes and a searching stare that could be disconcerting. She picked up immediately on my worries when I hinted that I could only use the softball game to promote the many social issues that surround transplantation, not Vanderbilt's program specifically, and certainly not myself.

"Or me," she said. "When we do interviews, there'll be no questions about what I'm doing, my latest record, anything like that. Not even my family. I want all exposure to be on those thousands of people in need of transplantation."

She involved me directly in the planning for the game with her business and PR people. It all reminded me of a particularly fast-paced and high-powered version of the Famous Bike Trip meetings at the hospital. I was no stranger to the moves she made to ensure that none of the celebrities had their egos inadvertently damaged by the detailed arrangements for transportation and accommodations and entertainment. University medical programs, too, had their share of status-conscious doctors, and entertainers had not cornered the market on egos. She was better at dealing with her celebrities, however, than I had ever been at handling medical stars.

We found each other's worlds fascinating, different as night and day. One evening on the West Coast, after she filmed a show, we visited to discuss the upcoming softball game. There was a whole slew of people in her suite talking the night away as Barbara and her friend and manager JoAnn Berry sat around eating peanuts and pizza, and drinking Cokes and staring their honest direct stares. All night, I tried to ask people what they did on the show, to get them to tell me in some technical detail of how the business worked, but I kept getting interrupted by questions about surgery, the kinds of cases we handled, who called the recipients when a donor was found, who flew off to pick up the hearts, how we got them beating again.

JoAnn handled Barbara's appearances on the talk shows and variety specials; she had done a thorough job of conveying our desires to the producers. It was evident by the kinds of questions the researcher from the "Today Show" asked when she called me at the hospital the day before we were to fly up to New York. She caught me between operations, in the locker room, and I was a bit self-conscious as I talked to her on the wall phone with my associates passing in and out, listening as they changed their scrubs. Not exactly what a surgeon usually does.

She asked very few questions about the game, but a number of well-informed ones on transplants. She was after the statistics: how many potential donors; how many real donors; how many patients need hearts; how many got them; how many died waiting; who could donate? Someone had tutored her well. And it paid off.

Phil Donahue was sitting in for Bryant Gumbel that day, and he apologized before we went on the air for not being more informed; he admitted that he was a little nervous. It seemed strange to me that someone of his visibility, accustomed to interviewing daily, would be nervous, but I guess we all become less at ease outside our familiar surroundings. But the interview went like clockwork, Barbara fielding the early questions about the game and then leading Donahue to direct his questions to me. And I got my organ-donor sound bites out to millions and millions of people I could not have reached in a lifetime of short drives and quick flights.

Larry King was a different matter. Immediately after we had finished the "Today Show," we took off for Washington. When we arrived at the studio, King was not to be seen. One of his assistants had a list of the questions he would ask. Barbara read them and turned white with anger. They were all about her, her accident, her career, her music, her museum. She looked up and said, "Nope."

"Nope?" asked the assistant.

"This ain't the interview we're doing," she said, putting on a deeper southern drawl than I'd ever heard her use.

"But, you've got to. These are the questions we rehearsed. These are the questions we made for Larry."

JoAnn took it from there. "You get the producer out here, now, or we're not gonna do the show," she said in no uncertain terms. The agreement had been that Barbara would appear with me and the topic would be transplantation; nothing else was acceptable. Yes, Barbara and JoAnn were committed to the cause; self-promotion was a nonissue. I got a real taste of why these two women were so successful—conviction, determination, and no room for compromise.

When the assistant hesitated, Barbara looked at me and said, "Dr. Frist, I'm sorry, and I really apologize. Les' go." I just wanted to say to Barbara to go ahead and do the show the way they wanted, that I did not need to be on it, that maybe she could just mention transplantation in passing. But, no way, she stuck to her guns.

The producer, a bit miffed by the disturbance, appeared and during the minute break before the interview told Larry King to throw out the interview. He winged it. It really threw me off my stride, great media star that I had become in twenty-four hours. But Barbara told him she loved him at the end. *A* for effort, I thought to myself.

I took it on the chin some for those two shows. Almost everywhere I went for the next month, it seemed as if somebody had something snide or witty to say about "Today" or Barbara or Larry or Phil. But there were dividends, and knowing that these dividends would pay off in helping others made it more than worth it. Several local shows picked up on the message. A couple of the news channels did pieces on transplantation and the Vanderbilt program, one following a heart-lung patient named Judy Williams through her long wait from the day she was listed through, we hoped, her operation and her life afterward. And a local talk show invited me on.

I was an old pro by this time, and I took my own star with me, Mark Johnson. He drove up to Nashville for the event, and I met him at the station. I did what Barbara had done to me and shifted all the questions toward Mark. He handled them quite well. Mark's thick black eyebrows would bob, and he'd flash his boyish smile and talk about deer hunting, and the host would almost fall over in his chair.

"Does it bother you?"

I would not have known what the guy meant, but Mark picked up on it right away.

"To have someone else's heart? No. I don't think about it. I'm just grateful to have the life I'm living, the life I never thought I would have. I look forward with great joy to the next forty or fifty years of my life, just like anyone else my age."

"Dr. Frist," the host said, "how do you help these patients most?"

"Well, in transplantation the surgeon doesn't play all that big a role. It's like being a good mechanic. I guess the way you help your patients—you help them in ways you can't really tell. The other night I saw a sixty-three-year-old patient waiting for a heart. I said to him what Mark just said, 'You are only sixty-three, and that is very young, and you have a long healthy life ahead of you.' And he said to me, 'You know, my world over the last six months has been collapsing around me and nothing could go right. I was told I was going to die, I'd never see my wife again, I'd not be able to have hobbies. Then you said a simple thing, you said that I have a long healthy life ahead of me. That statement made every-thing seem right all of a sudden. It gave me hope.' I hardly even remember saying it to the guy, but you see how even the smallest things can have a tremendous impact."

"Is that right, Mark? Is that how he helped you?"

"No," Mark said. "He gave me a new heart."

We all laughed.

Afterward, I took Mark out to dinner with Karyn and me, and we had a wonderful time going back over the show and listening to him describe the ups and downs of a newlywed transplant. He mentioned that he had ridden his motorcycle up from Knoxville and had a close call, forced onto the interstate median by a sixteen-wheeler.

"You have to watch that," I said.

"Oh, Bill," Karyn said. "Can't you stop being his doctor for just one night?"

"I am his doctor," I said. "I can't help it. But that's not what I meant, anyway. You have to watch those motorcycles. I had a bad accident in high school on one when I was just about a year younger than you, and I almost died."

"Did you sign a donor card?" Mark asked.

We all laughed.

As I paid the bill, I noticed Karyn looking at me strangely. Had I said something wrong? Later, it seemed a premonition.

4

I'll never forget that day.

It was exactly a week before Jimmy Moore's Famous Bike Ride.

That morning, I dropped in to see Jim and Shirley Hayes at the cooperative-care unit.

Many of our long-term care and cancer patients stayed in the cooperative-care unit, separated from the main hospital building but still part of the medical center. The rooms were large and had a few amenities—a chair, couch, and table, for example—but a nurse was on duty twenty-four hours a day. Shirley could spend all day there with Jim and not have to deal with the inconveniences of visiting-hours regulations and the stream of nurses, residents, and doctors that had swarmed around him back on the regular ward. Still, it was a far cry from the halfway house, even a further cry from home, and Jim never left his room except to visit me or Walter or Jay Groves down in rehab.

Jim was steadily improving and we had just about run the full course of the radiation treatment. I had hopes. His memory remained a problem, though it too was getting better. Most of the time now he could remember his son's name, and he no longer confused me with Dr. Baumgartner, who had performed his first transplant. He was having trouble reading, learning the basics all over again, and it frustrated him. There was nothing wrong with his eyes, so we assumed it was the effect of the virus. Hour upon hour, Shirley would patiently read to him from the newspaper or from various books, novels and nonfiction, that she bought him or borrowed from one of us.

Shirley had, in fact, become his alter ego. When he did have difficulty remembering something, she would carefully fill in the blanks for him. She was at the point where she could anticipate when he was coming upon a blank and gently prepare him before he grew angry racking his brain. She could complete his sentences, knowing exactly what he intended to say. But she was beginning to show signs of wear and tear.

And now Jim's four-year-old son, in addition to his teenage daughter, was beginning to react to the long, doubt-filled separation from his parents and display signs of emotional disturbance. He had reversed his toilet training and refused to eat almost everything. They were thinking about therapy, but unlike Jim's medical treatment—which was covered by the federal government (after a long battle during his first transplant) as part of Jim's veteran's benefits—they had no third-party insurer to pay the costs. In addition, Shirley had just been informed by her boss at the Post Office in Knoxville that she was being let go. For half a year she had gotten by on compassionate leave, then she took a six-month leave of absence. The postal service said it would make every effort to find her a job when she could go back to work.

Through it all, though, she had never left Jim's side, and she did not intend to. She had prepared all his meals when they had lived across the street, and she was still giving Jim his medicines and keeping his patient charts, taking him to physical therapy each day, becoming almost as sophisticated as our program's nurses in caring for him and watching out for his health. Jim's situation provided yet another perfect example of transplantation in general, the need for a good, solid, supportive mate, one who really meant "in sickness and in health," because he or she would certainly come to understand all that phrase can mean.

"Hi, Dr. Frist," Jim said. "How's it going?"

"Fine," I said. "You are coming along just perfectly. But I really stopped by to give you some good news. You asked me about the bicycle trip—"

"You don't think he's well enough to do that?" Shirley said, clearly concerned. "Do you?"

"No. No, I don't. But it's next weekend, and I'm going to fly down to Knoxville on Sunday. It starts Friday night, but I have to go to a transplant meeting out in California, and I don't know if I can get back in time. But the reason I bring it up: I thought maybe the two of you might like to fly down with me. In my plane. Maybe see your family for the day. Then fly back with me that afternoon. You're too fragile to discharge from the hospital, but I can risk sneaking you out for half a day. Can't tell anyone. It's our secret mission."

"You mean it?" Jim said.

"I sure do," I said.

"You know how to fly one of them things?" Shirley asked suspiciously.

"Yes," I said. "But I probably won't be flying this plane. I'll have someone take us."

"Just how big a plane is it?"

"Who cares, Shirley," Jim said. "I get to see little Jimmy."

Shirley looked at me shyly under her dark eyebrows. "I never been in one of them little planes. But I guess you do everything once when you get married to Jim Hayes."

Jim thought that was about the funniest thing she had ever said.

Back in my office, there was a note to call Patricia Smith.

Though I did not recognize the name, my secretary Faye had written across the note "Al Moore's secretary." Little warning lights were going off in my head as I dialed the number.

"This is weird," said Patricia Smith. "You don't know me, and maybe it's none of my business. But something's wrong, Dr. Frist. I went into his office this morning—into Al's office, I mean—and he was just sitting there, slumped back sort of in his chair, his feet propped up, with what you call a vacant stare in his eyes. I mean, it's not like him. He said he had a hangover, and like I said, maybe it's none of my business, but I'm worried about him, so I thought I'd call."

"You did the right thing," I said. "Is Al there now?"

"No, he's over at the courthouse."

"Would you do something for me?" I asked. "Would you have him call me or Jan, my nurse, the minute he gets back? And if he won't call, would you call me back?"

"Yes, I will do that," she said soberly.

241

"And—"

"Yes?"

"Will you stay there until Al returns, and if he doesn't come back also call me? We might have to go over to the courthouse looking for him."

What did I do that afternoon?

It's blank. Nothing. Nothing important.

Around four o'clock that afternoon Al got through to me, and I quickly shut off his tale about losing sleep and being tired from the night before, which escalated then to having a drink or two.

"Al," I said, "have you been missing your medicines?"

"Dr. Frist, I tell you, it's just a hangover. I know what a hangover feels like."

"Have you missed taking your medicines? Even once?"

"Just last night. Lizzy, my girlfriend, and I—I'll be honest with you. I had a little too much to drink; I forgot."

"You forgot?"

"I was in the throes of passion, if you know what I mean," he laughed.

"How many times?"

"Dr. Frist. You sound like that federal judge. I've got a new heart. The rest of me is still thirty-five years old. We only did—"

"This is not something to joke about. How many times have you missed your immunosuppressants?"

"I told you. Once." He paused. I waited. "Twice. Once last night. A week ago. Thursday, I think."

"I want you to come on over here, right now," I said. "I want you to come to the emergency room and see the cardiologist on duty. I'll call him. His name is—, hold on." I asked Faye to find out who was on duty. "I'll give you his name in a minute. I want you to describe your symptoms to him exactly. Don't lie and don't interpret. Don't say it's a hangover. I have a case to do right now, but I'll be by before he's done with you if I can. In any event, don't leave the hospital until I talk to you."

So I had a case. I operated on someone. I got there later than I intended.

The cardiologist. He was smiling. Al had obviously told him about the night before, played up my worry, played down the danger.

"Your patient is fine," the cardiologist said, slapping me on the back. "He's got a little cold. Simple virus. Nothing we should be overly concerned about. His temperature is up just a bit. A degree above normal, and I'm not even sure if it's that high. I'd say he's had a little too much fun."

"We need to do an emergency biopsy right now," I said.

"Well, if you think that's necessary."

"I want a room ready for him tonight when I'm done. He's not to leave this hospital until we get the results of the biopsy."

"I'll see to it," the doctor said coldly.

Al had to break his date with Lizzy. Six hours later, he had developed full-blown rejection, confirmed by his biopsy. He could hardly breathe. We gave him a bolus of steroids. He was hours away from dying.

It was midnight when Jan caught up with me.

She was paler than I had seen her since Jean Lefkowitz had died. She stood looking at me. Not speaking.

"Don't worry," I smiled. "He'll pull through. He was stupid, but it won't happen again. I think he's learned his lesson."

"Who?" Jan said, bewildered.

"Al. Al Moore."

"You haven't heard," she said.

"Haven't heard?"

"Dr. Frist, it's Mark Johnson. He's dead."

"Dead?"

She nodded. "It was an accident. A hunting accident."

"When?"

"This morning in a field near his home. He died before they could get him to a hospital."

Four in the morning. Another sleepless night.

I had gone home depressed, told Karyn, and we talked. She

could not forget the dinner we had with him last week. The night we went on television. How he had said he was looking forward to the next fifty years of life. How I had warned him to be careful on his motorcycle and talked about my accident in high school. She had never heard me tell anyone else about it. And then I thought, I have to get back. Somebody will tell Al Moore. I have to make sure they don't tell Al Moore.

I came in at five and talked to Holley.

"C'mon, Dr. Frist," she said, "I'm not that stupid. I wouldn't tell Al anything like that. I couldn't. I wouldn't know what to say. I can't believe it anyway. It's just not fair. We do everything right and . . . Al's fine. He has been sleeping like a baby, especially after his girlfriend left."

"His girlfriend?"

"Yeah, Lizzy. She's something else. Honey blond and wow. She's a nice little girl. She sat all night outside his room. She just left. Went home to change so she'd look good when he wake—"

"I don't want her in there."

"She—"

"I don't want her in there. Sleeping in the room or anything like that. She is complicating his recovery."

"He wants to see her," Holley said.

"Fine. She can visit him. But I don't want her staying in the room. I should talk to her."

"She's scared out of her wits."

"I need to talk to her and tell her the seriousness of this situation."

"She said she'd be back at six," Holley said, and walked away. Ticked. OK. The girl as well as Al had to know what one careless night might mean

Six in the morning. She stands there, her short hair not spiked but set and she looks young, too young, and her big blue eyes grow bigger and rounder as I tell her that Al is suffering from severe rejection and if we had not gotten to him when we did he might be dead now. Her lower lip begins to tremble when I tell her that he will have to stay in the hospital for at least a week and that he is not a man who can be careless. Her whole frame begins to shake and she drops back against the wall as I say that every time he lights up a cigarette or drinks liquor and forgets to take his medicine he's running the same risk that it will happen again only next time we might not be so lucky and he would die before we got to him. And she is crying openly now when I say that at least he seems to understand that better and so should she if she's going to continue seeing him and the crowd around the desk keeps looking over our way as Lizzy shakes and cries and I bear down harder thinking

I can never tell enough people who need to know all the ins and outs and ups and downs and what does it matter anyway because no matter what you do somebody you have never seen comes along and puts a bullet through Mark Johnson and calls it an accident though who knows because he was taking steroids and maybe they affected his concentration and he just got careless but that's just the surgeon in you who always wants to accept responsibility and take

Control. Take control of yourself. I wasn't proud of the way I'd treated Lizzy. It wasn't her I was angry at, of course, but Al, and not Al, really, but Mark Johnson, and not Mark either, but death itself. I was standing in the bathroom next to the scrub lockers on the third floor, looking at myself in the mirror. I could imagine tears welling up in my eyes, their steamy feel as my vision became blurred, but it never happened. I could imagine doubling up my fists and striking the walls or the metallic hand dryer and just screaming at the top of my lungs, "It's not fair. It's not fair. It's not fair."

But I didn't do it.

5

I spent a lot of that next week in the lab, implanting the new test model of the LVAD in sheep, trying to perfect a mechanical heart that met all of Shumway's requirements. From time to time I read in the paper about the movement against animal research, and I sympathized, wanting to agree that there was some better way. But my experience had taught me it was the only way to learn. All of Shumway's breakthroughs had come through animal research. To progress at all in modern medicine we simply had to bounce back and forth between the lab, clinical application, and the lab again, asking questions based on clinical problems based in turn on patients, setting up hypotheses, testing them experimentally, finding the answer, saving the patient.

That week it also helped me work through the blues.

I left on Thursday for Los Angeles, where I would see all the folks from Stanford again and maybe escape the doldrums. Before I headed for the airport, I sat in on our weekly transplant meeting, which we held at the crack of dawn each Thursday of every week.

When I arrived at Vanderbilt, I instituted the meetings so everyone on the transplant team could discuss any and all issues on a regular basis. By everyone, I meant the surgeons, the social workers, the psychiatrists, the nurses, the scheduling secretary, the hospital ethicists, the chaplain, the admissions officer, the immunologists who did the tissue typing, the coordinators from the procurement agency, surgical residents, and medical students who happened to be on the service at the time.

We met at seven in the morning, a civilized hour by a surgeon's clock, but rather early for some of the others. No one openly complained, and few ever missed the discussions, which ranged from the weekly review of transplant patients' progress to the ethical dilemmas of allocating scarce resources—not just the organs, but the funds for treatment, too. Everyone participated, everyone made his or her contribution. And it was essential that they did. Social worker Janie Webb's comment that she was having difficulty finding telephone service for Jay Gregory was just as important to the program as surgical resident Ed Gerhardt's concerns about his difficulty in treating Arthur Murphy's life-threatening aspergillus lung infection.

The twenty of us sat at a long, narrow table munching donuts and drinking coffee as we reviewed the lists that documented the program's activities. On the first page appeared data on each of the recipients: name, hospital record number, date of transplant, age at operation, the ailment that brought them to us in the first place, the date the transplant was performed, and date and results of the last biopsy. On the second page, we scanned the eight patients who were on the active waiting list, some at home now, some in the hospital, wearing their beepers, worrying about the fateful call. After that appeared the names and the essential facts about twenty-two patients referred to us in the past six months as possible candidates for heart and heart-lung transplants.

Page one: Douglas Goodwin, a sixty-one-year-old man from nearby Franklin topped the first list. He was still coming to the office twice a week, but six weeks out from his transplant, he was progressing well in his rehab program with Jay Groves. He walked on the treadmill for forty-five minutes a day four days a week—not bad for a man who had been hospitalized eleven times in the past year for recurring heart failure, a man many might consider too old to transplant.

Next came Velma Johnson, a delightful forty-year-old black woman we had operated on six months earlier. When I thought about Velma, I pictured her—before she got her new heart—in the intensive-care unit, where she lived for two months. She suffered recurring episodes of sudden death, a term we use to describe her heart's tendency to fibrillate suddenly and stop pumping. At least twice a week a nurse called a stat code, and the emergency code team rushed in to shock her heart back to life. We finally found her a heart. Now, she was at home and happy.

I came to Mark Johnson's name. It was painful just reading it off the sheet. It appeared that week for the last time, with "Died" typed next to last Friday's date where the biopsy information was usually recorded.

We all knew by then what happened, so I talked briefly about the funeral arrangements for anyone who wanted to go. If Mark's heart had caused his death, pathologist Jim Atkinson would have performed an autopsy and studied the heart in detail. Jim would then have shared his findings with us in a formal slide presentation, and we would also have studied the case to figure out how to treat recipients better in the future. But not today. Mark's heart had not caused his death.

So we all avoided the subject and talked for a while about Jimmy Moore's Famous Bike Trip and the Mandrell celebrity softball game. I described the special "Meet the Stars" rally at the Vanderbilt Plaza Hotel before the game. Hesitating to mention the price because few people around the table could afford to go, I softly said, "Tickets are one hundred dollars apiece," and quickly added, "but it all goes to the program."

"Which reminds me," said Janie Webb, our social worker, "I don't know if you've thought about this, but how is Jonathan going to get to the game? They don't have a car, and I don't think his mom should have to pay for a taxicab. She might not do it anyway and try something silly like walking over."

"We'll pay the taxi," I said. "Jan, can you see to it? You might check with Mandrell's people. Maybe they'll even want to send a limousine. She's sure crazy about him. Did you see the poster?"

"Yeah," Walter said. "He looks great, sitting right there in the center. A real charmer."

"That's why I always use his slide in my talks. Anything else, Janie?"

"Well, I'm a bit worried about Jullie Haynes. Seems to be some kind of tension there in the family. Jullie's mother and father are divorced. It's her mother and Jullie's husband who are staying

248

with her all the time. She hasn't seen her father since she was sixteen, and now he says he wants to come down from Utah or something. And she says she won't let him in her room. The mother swears he's on his way anyway. I mean, I think she's already depressed, with that other girl's death—what was her name? Belinda Moreau. And then Jullie waited so long for the transplant. And they've got no money."

"I'll talk to her when I get back," I said. "What do you think? Can we keep him away?"

"Out of the room, certainly," Walter said.

"But out of the hospital?"

"We don't need any scenes in the waiting room. It's tense enough in there already."

Janie's comments about money reminded me that Jullie's payments for her hospitalization had not been completely resolved. "What about the money, Janice?" Janice Jett handled the financial arrangements for our patients. "Anything?"

"She doesn't qualify for Medicaid. The money Belinda Moreau wanted to give her is still tied up in the estate, and it wouldn't be near enough anyway."

"Uh-oh," said Jim Atkinson. "Looks like we swallow another one."

"You can't keep doing this, Dr. Frist," Janice said. "We still have problems with almost all insurance companies on heart-lungs; they still regard them as experimental. And the way the new Medicaid rules are set up, even if they did pay, you're bound to lose money on each operation, because it costs us like $89,000, and Medicaid for just hearts reimburses only $39,000. We're supposed to make it up on paying patients, but there seems to be very few of them coming in the doors."

"Give me your tired, your poor, your sick at heart," Atkinson said, and everyone groaned.

Keep the meeting moving. Randy Atkins, twenty-one years old, was doing well. Randy had received his new heart seven years ago at Stanford. He came to us from his Kentucky home the year before for his annual visit. It was easier for him to cross state lines to see us than to trek back to California each year. Randy liked Nashville so much that he quit his job, moved to the city, and found work, of all places, in the pharmacy right here at Vanderbilt Hospital.

Walter, seeing that we were running out of time, brought up an issue I was hoping to avoid, especially since the ethicists were sitting in force around the table.

"Hey," Walter said. "What about this AIDS thing?"

"AIDS?" ten voices said at once.

I looked at Walter and whispered, "Thanks a lot.

"Guess we better discuss it. We got AIDS right here in River City. A fellow, needs a transplant, called us from California. He's HIV-III positive, which means he is carrying the AIDS virus. He is doing well clinically from the standpoint of the virus, totally asymptomatic, but his heart is failing. Apparently he got the virus from a blood transfusion years ago, but his history is not entirely clear to me. One center refused to list him. But, it's even more complicated than that. He told me that the center tested him without his written consent. So, he's suing the hospital, claiming their intrusion into his privacy now prevents his being accepted into a transplant program. And he wants to know if we'll take him."

There was utter silence.

It was a problem we hadn't had to face before.

"Jan," I said, "do we have everybody who comes in sign a consent form before we test for AIDS?"

"I think so. We test everybody. They cannot be admitted to the hospital without signing the consent to be tested," she said.

I remembered well last year's heated meetings in which we worked out the hospital's policy. Doing the testing, though, did not resolve the tragedy before us. Realizing that we could not solve the complex issues in a few minutes, I set up a special committee composed of Jan, Walter, an infectious-disease specialist, the hospital chaplain, and an ethicist to determine whether or not we should accept patients who harbored the AIDS virus.

Next on the list: patient James Bunning, a forty-three-year-old go-getter who lived near Chicago and who managed a chain of eight hotels, not slowed down a bit by his new heart. It had taken him some time after his transplant, though, to convince potential bosses that a transplant recipient could perform well on the job.

And Charles Mullins had returned to work as an agricultural researcher for the University of Tennessee. Fourteen-year-old Robbie Brickner was back at school and so was thirteen-year-old Corey Pachmayr. Dennis Warren, fifty-five, had just returned for a biopsy this week, having spent the past six weeks on a nation-wide tour with his wife.

And so it went. Down the list with each patient. We reviewed the biopsies, any recent observations in the clinic, and social problems. I then described our work in the lab with the LVAD and finished with, "I think we'll be doing total implants within two years." Either that stunned everyone into silence, or they were too tired by the long meeting to speak.

When I got to Jim Hayes, I turned to Walter for his report.

"He came to clinic Tuesday," Walter said, grinning from ear to ear. "Just walked in big as life and sat down and started talking. I know he's still got several more radiation treatments scheduled, but he looks great. To see him, you'd never know he was sick a day in his life. A walking miracle man."

Heads shook in amazement.

Page Two: We closed the meeting with a brief review of the patients who were waiting for transplantation. I hoped and prayed that we would find hearts for all eight of them. But I knew we would not. Two of the eight would in all likelihood die before we found hearts. As I read the names, I wondered which two I would lose. It pushed me to give more talks, to educate more physicians, and to be thankful for the help of the media and people like Barbara Mandrell. Someday, I hoped to look at eight names and be confident all eight would make it.

* * *

251

The hotel in Los Angeles was a monster built on the back lot of one of the old studios—Universal, I think. The place was filled with surgeons, every prominent heart surgeon in the world except for Denton Cooley and Ed Stinson. With so many surgeons, the hotel staff was miserable, learning the kind of patience it took to be a nurse as grown men cut in line, stormed into roped-off areas, sat in closed restaurants, and refused to abandon overcrowded meeting rooms.

Two of the talks that afternoon intrigued me. One was by Dr. Joel Cooper from Toronto, who had been having some success with double-lung transplants. The operations had received bad press that resembled that of heart transplants in the early days. Hardly anyone was doing them, and people were skeptical of the results being reported at this meeting. I shared that skepticism to a degree, though I kept thinking about Shumway's seven stages in the acceptance of a new surgical therapy.

The second was a panel discussion on anencephalic babies, which made me think of both Jonathan Jones and Nancy Davis, the organ coordinator who went with Rusty and me to pick up Jim Hayes's third heart. Brain-death statutes in almost all the states had made the procedure for certifying death very specific and virtually error-free, with one exception. Anencephalic babies were born with a fatal neurologic anomaly, dead by all the brain-dead criteria save one, a slight activity in the brain stem. There was no hope for them; none would live. They had no real brain function when they were born, just enough spark to keep their bodies breathing till they could be put on a ventilator. If you took them off, they would lose even that tiny spark. But they could not be declared brain dead using the legal definitions.

Infants don't have automobile accidents. Few infants who died left transplantable organs. And the demand for such organs was large, around 400 to 500 a year. That was one reason why the decision to transplant Jonathan was difficult. Given the extreme rarity of an infant donor heart, surgeons simply didn't like to take any risks with unsuitable recipients. Three thousand anencephalic babies were born a year, enough to solve our demand

252

many times over—but we never used them. Occasionally a pregnant mother would go to term knowing her child was anencephalic, in order to donate the organs for transplantation. But
given the brain-death laws, a surgeon could not legally use the
organs. Doctors can't break the laws, even to save lives. And
legislators were loathe to change the law, because of the very real
possibility that it might seem to an ill-informed public that they
were trying to play God by taking organs from some newborns
and giving them to others.

I saw Vaughn Starnes across the room during the session and
caught up with him afterward. We met his wife, Janet, and
headed off for a reunion, cocktails for some, a much needed snack
for others.

"What did you think about the discussion?" I asked.

"Interesting," Vaughn said. "I never know what to make of it.
Another transplant tempest in a tea pot. They're dead. They've
got good hearts. We should use them."

"I know," I said. "One of the coordinators back in Nashville,
Nancy Davis, was dealing with a couple. In the seventh month of
pregnancy they tell the wife her child is anencephalic. She and
her husband talk and they decide to carry the baby to term in
order to donate, so they approach Nancy. She agrees with the
couple, applauds what they are trying to do, but she simply
cannot legally help them. She plays around with the idea of
advising them to go ahead, donate the organs, find a doctor who
will take the risk, and challenge the law to get it changed. But she
does not want to commit a crime."

"Nobody does," Vaughn said.

It occurred to me that by refusing to face the issue, we were
allowing living babies to die by legal default.

"You did a baby, right?" Janet asked.

I smiled. "Little Jonathan Jones. Barbara Mandrell wants to
make him a star."

"You're the star," Janet said.

"Yeah," Vaughn added. "We caught your 'Today Show' song
and dance."

"I almost didn't do Jonathan because of his family's difficult financial situation. Lots of potential social problems. Then I did and he had some bradycardia post-op. I went ahead and put in a pacemaker, although he never uses it now. But he's doing fine."

"You remember my baby?" Vaughn said.

"Who could forget?"

The case was famous at Stanford. Shumway even used it in the funniest presidential address anyone ever gave at the American Association of Thoracic Surgeons.

Vaughn did the actual operation, but Ed Stinson retrieved the heart. It was three days before Christmas in 1986. Stanford was notified of a four-month-old heart donor in Fargo, North Dakota, whose blood type and weight matched perfectly a five-month-old recipient in critical care, dying of endocardial fibroelastosis. It would take anywhere from four to five hours, which was too long, but Shumway decided to go ahead, given the paucity of infant hearts.

Stinson and six others chartered a Lear jet and flew 2,000 miles into the North Dakota tundra carrying their usual surgical gear and dressed in their California scrub suits and white coats. They got there with no trouble and found that the heart was sound. A team from Minnesota took the liver, then Stinson removed the heart, put it in cold storage, and high-stepped back to the waiting Lear.

One of the engines would not start. Precious minutes ticked by as the gang got out giant hair dryers and tried to warm up the engine. No such luck. They rammed a burning broom into the mouth of the jet. Nothing happened. They deplaned, and Stinson requested an audience with the colonel in charge of the North Dakota Air National Guard. He asked for a supersonic jet to blast them into the heart of Palo Alto. The colonel patiently explained that his job was to protect the north-central United States from a surprise attack by the Russians, not ferry a bunch of crazy, thinly clad surgeons into the land of dreams.

Stinson was desperate. He called the governor of North Dakota and asked him to pull rank on the colonel and release a jet. Two and a half hours had elapsed. The governor gave the colonel the order, and Stinson and company got an F-4 Phantom. The F-4 is a two-passenger supersonic jet with a range of one thousand miles. A pilot fits, and a navigator, but there is no other storage area that is temperature and pressure controlled. The navigator would have to hold the ice chest containing the donor heart on his lap.

"Wait a minute," he said. "If I have to eject, that thing will go right through me. No way. No thank you." The pilot flew solo, the chest lashed to the seat next to him, stopping briefly to refuel in Ogden, Utah. Undaunted, Vaughn had already started to open up the recipient's chest. He was ready at 4:15 Pacific Standard Time. The heart made it by 5:30. The run took eight hours, but the heart survived. Two weeks later, the infant was discharged and the child continued to do well today. Stinson and his comrades caught a commercial flight back to San Francisco, arriving long after the operation was over.

"There is something else I'm doing at Vanderbilt that will interest you in particular, Vaughn, and Janet as well," I said.

Janet looked over. Vaughn said, "Oh?"

"I'm working on a task force at Vanderbilt on the residency programs. We're going to try to change the way medicine is taught."

"Never happen," Vaughn said. It was somewhat of a sore subject between him and his wife. Vaughn's residency, like that of so many of us, had been hard on them as a couple. Every other night in the hospital for five years simply does not make sense. It's not normal and it's not healthy. It's a tradition that was begun long ago and has been perpetuated without justification, to my way of reasoning.

"What are you going to do?" Janet asked.

"Well, you know there's this whole movement for reform, not very popular among the older surgeons, within the Accreditation Council for Graduate Medical Education, and I've been working on it there, too."

"I didn't know you were involved," Vaughn said.

"We're going to put the whole emphasis on education, not slave labor. So, one of the points in particular we're hitting hard is working conditions. On-call quarters and library resources have got to be adequate, of course, but so do basic support services like obtaining lab results easily. No more having residents spend an inordinate amount of time, nights, weekends, doing what secretaries or orderlies should be doing. Is it really necessary having a physician with twenty years of training behind him pushing patients around for their next tests, starting IVs, and drawing blood when there should be ancillary personnel doing these tasks? And the amount of time, the working hours, can't be the be-all and end-all of residency."

"Good luck," Vaughn said. "I don't believe it, but good luck."

"It's going to happen."

"You always were the optimist. Hospitals just aren't going to shell out the money. Residency has always been a cost-saving scam."

"We've got to change," I said. "We can't keep putting out surgical automatons. We need people who can think, too, about something other than a timely stitch well sewed. And who can spend some time with their families."

"Like me and you."

Now he had me started, so I wanted to finish my speech. "Both Massachusetts and New York have proposals on the books that would put a limit of eighty hours on the number of hours a week a resident could work. That would be a marked improvement. I think residents should be allowed one day a week away from the hospital, but few program directors are likely to let this happen. In addition, residents should be on call no more than every third night and clearly should be given some opportunity to rest after a twenty-four hour stint. It's a labor issue, but it is a patient-care issue as well."

Vaughn replied, "You are dreaming. You will never change the system."

"Vaughn, do you think the real world, those people outside of hospitals, who have regular, nonmedical jobs, those people who are patients as well, have any idea of what residents are forced to go through in their ritualistic process to become doctors? I mean, would you go through it again?"

Vaughn stopped. He and Janet exchanged glances.

"You mean," he said, "if I knew what I'd be doing now? If I had to go through residency again to have the kind of life we're leading now, would I do it?"

"Yes," I said.

"No way," he said, deadly serious. "Would you?"

I thought about it. Life was full of so many other alternatives, most of which had some degree of sanity.

"No," I said quietly, "I don't think I would." But the system can be changed.

The gang was all there at the grand cocktail reception that night in the hotel's glitzy, Hollywoodish ballroom. There was quite a spread and excellent wine, and Norman Shumway was in top form, talking about the future of transplantation coming down to a single pill. "You get your new heart, then a glass of water and this pill, about the size of a pearl say, and pop! in the mouth, no more rejection. Ever. Stinson's working on it," he said. "So it's a done thing. Hope for the walking dead."

Phil Oyer was there, too, talking to the guy who made Stanford's RATG in his garage. They were going over the ins and outs of incorporating, mass-producing the stuff. "Success would ruin you," I heard Oyer say as I walked up and shook his big, brawny hand. "Bill Frist. How's the easy life?"

Outside lay the City of Angels, but I was back at Stanford.

I bumped into Bill Baumgartner at the conference and, naturally enough, told him all about Jim Hayes. Later that night I called Karyn and told her to pack her bags, I was coming home early. We were going to make the opening day of Jimmy Moore's Famous Bike Trip. Then I called Jan.

"How's our boy Al doing?"

"Fine," Jan said. "He's feeling a lot better and his biopsy shows the rejection is clearing up. Dr. Merrill thinks he could go home if you want him to. Al certainly wants out. He's been asking me about the bike trip."

"No," I said. "No way. Absolutely not. In fact, I think I'll keep

257

him a few extra days, at least until I can get back and see him again."

"Are you laying it on a little thick on purpose?"

"You got me. This is our chance. We need to scare him a little, put the fear of God in him, let him feel how serious all this is."

"I understand," Jan said.

"Oh," I said, "Don't fret. He told me just last week, 'Dr. Frist, you can lie to me any time.' Only, I'm not lying. I'm maximizing this learning opportunity."

Ed Stinson was not at the conference, so after I rang off with Jan, I called him at home again for the first time in six months. It was getting to be a habit.

"Ed, this is Bill. Bill Frist."

"Bill," he said, the tone as well as the words exactly the same as six months ago. "Nice to hear from you. Where are you?"

"I'm in Los Angeles. At the transplant conference. I'm calling you to tell you about Jim Hayes," I said. "'Our' treatment worked."

Being Ed, he wanted the specifics. And being Ed, not once in the entire conversation that followed did he ask me about the conference attended by men and women he had worked with all his life. Not even about the weather.

6

The old couple leaned over and whispered to the little boy, then gestured toward our group as the lobby doors of the small private airport closed on the whine of revving jet engines. Even at this distance I could see the puzzled look on the boy's face. There was his mother, but who was the strange man she was holding on to, the funny man with a stick and that blue thing, like an outlaw, over his face? Then he recognized his dad and came flying across the room in quick short steps, a miniature imitation of his father's walk, and leaped up high into Jim Hayes's arms.

It was Sunday morning. I had gotten back from California early enough Friday for Karyn and me to fly over to Johnson City, stay with the troops in a motel on the edge of town Friday night, and see them off Saturday morning.

We helped Jay Groves check them over, making sure their chest monitors worked and their blood pressures and temperatures were normal. And we had watched as the PR folks from Equicor struggled to get the huge sign with the company's name atop the four-wheel-drive land wagon that carried the extra bicycles and all the medical equipment. As they stuck their adhesive signs onto each of the cars that would follow them across the state, I heard Jimmy Moore mumbling about how this had gotten away from the original purpose of the event: donor awareness.

But he was happy enough the next morning in Bristol, which sits half in Virginia and half in Tennessee. The town's two mayors saw the gang off, declaring it Donor Awareness Day in both townships and releasing a thousand balloons, donor cards attached, that drifted up high and away into the strong winds of a gloomy sky that promised rain. Karyn and I followed them in a truck I had borrowed from the desk clerk at the airport the night before when the rental car I ordered had not shown up. We took photographs of them all, Jimmy, and Jan, and Jeff Myers, a kidney-transplant patient, and the girls from Equicor and Nashville's organ-procurement agency, with Ron Wynn valiantly bringing up the rear. Then we flew back Saturday night for an evening with the kids.

Sunday morning I picked up Jim and Shirley at the cooperative-care unit and headed off to Knoxville. As Jim Hayes and his family walked off to spend a precious four hours at home, I invited the old ramrod pilot who had been flying me around for a month to join me at Knoxville's city park for the arrival of my bike-mad patients and coworkers. To my surprise, the taciturn fellow accepted. He seemed to enjoy himself as the local organ-procurement coordinator rushed about in the heat of a bright summer day orchestrating the growing crowd and the camera crews in anticipation of the big moment. And before long they came puffing into view, surrounded by a score of local bicyclers, a few of them also organ-transplant patients, Jimmy's beet-red, sun- and wind-burned face leading the pack.

There were speeches galore. The coordinator for the regional organ-procurement agency who had organized the event welcomed everybody. The president of Equicor's PR firm gave his pitch, a little chagrined at losing his huge metal cartop sign to the winds and traffic of east Tennessee highways, much to Jimmy Moore's delight. I spoke briefly, being careful to thank Equicor for its financial and organizational support and for being in the forefront of insurance agencies in covering all transplants. Then each of the three patients spoke in turn. As the crowd began to cheer, there was Jimmy, jumping back up to the microphone, shouting, "Organ-donor cards! Don't forget the organ-donor cards!"

After, the group stood around while Jay Groves checked them and their bicycle equipment and the local news conducted interviews. I could see the three of them falling into categories for the media: Jimmy Moore, serious, athletic, inspiring, articulate; Ron Wynn, black, funny, touching; Jeff Myers, young, naive, the heartthrob of the group. In time I rescued Jan from the crowd to take her back to Nashville with me that afternoon. She would join up with the group again on Wednesday when they reached Nashville.

Right now I needed Jan to interview a prospective patient with me while we were in Knoxville. Marvin Lee was a nineteen-year-old black man who was dying from a congenital heart ailment that had plagued him throughout his life. Knowing that he desperately needed a transplant, but that his parents did not have much money, I had arranged to see them at the private airport in Knoxville on Sunday afternoon to save them the expense of a trip to Vanderbilt.

"Back to work," I said, grinning.

"We're flying back in that plane you rented?" she asked, looking sideways at the pilot over talking to Ron.

"That's right," I said.

"Just how small is it?"

"Oh, no," I laughed. "Not you, too."

I had never seen her blush before. Maybe it was the sun.

Nightly, I watched the cyclists' progress across the state on the television at home or in the office, calling up images of the map of Tennessee like those used on "That's Incredible!" and drawing in my mind that mysterious black line moving past route numbers and city names. As I predicted, the media could have cared less about any of the country wilderness between towns and only picked them up a few miles outside of each station. That was okay, because it gave the gang an opportunity to ride in the motor vehicles without losing face when Jay decided they were too exhausted or the weather turned bad. Ron Wynn did a lot of driving that week and took a lot of kidding for it, which I thought was good for him. It might even get him to pay more serious attention to his weight. They hit Nashville at noon on Wednesday, smack dab in the middle of National Secretary's Day.

Legislative Plaza was filled with young women in their light summer dresses and middle-aged women in business suits who were a little nonplussed when the troops came tooling up on their bikes surrounded by camera crews and trucks. They took over the secretaries' podium to give transplant pep talks. And the women cheered gamely.

That night the governor threw a huge cocktail party in the boys' honor at his mansion, which I did not attend. Walter represented Vanderbilt. I had already taken too much grief for my appearances with Barbara Mandrell, on the "Today Show," and with Larry King. I didn't know for sure she would be there, but with the softball game not far off, I did not see how she could afford to miss the opportunity to promote it, and I figured I'd just keep the proverbial low profile.

I heard it went well from Walter—and his wife, Morgan—who flew out to Memphis with Karyn and me on Saturday for the grand finale. Phil Brodnax, an old high-school chum who had moved to Memphis and become a wheeler-dealer, met us at the airport in a stretch limo. We had a delightful brunch at the elegant Peabody Hotel, where those famous ducks march daily through the lobby. Walter and I both found it difficult to explain that we simply couldn't drive up to the rally in a limo to greet several bone-tired, self-sacrificing heart-transplant patients in such a style. We parked the limousine blocks away behind a clump of trees and hiked to the city museum where a large crowd had gathered to welcome the lads.

Half the crowd were transplant patients, wearing white T-shirts with big red letters proclaiming the fact. Many of the others wore similar T-shirts with blue letters that said Be an Organ Donor. The Baptist Hospital's transplant team was there, as were two local surgeons who specialized in liver transplants. They spoke along with the regulars, but the last word went to Ron and Jimmy.

The joking stopped as Ron talked about how people always asked him if it bothered him that he had someone else's heart, and he said he was going to shout what he always felt like shouting: "NO! THIS IS MY HEART! Not that I'm not grateful, you understand, because I know if it wasn't for the kindness and the love of a stranger who thought enough to give, I wouldn't be here. A lot of people have called us heroes this week, but the real heroes are those people, the ones who donate their organs so that out of their tragic deaths people like me can have a life."

"I've heard a lot about heroes, too, this week," said a very tired Jimmy Moore, standing at the top of the museum steps and looking out over us and beyond. "I want to tell you about some of

262

my heroes. My heroes are all those who were on the list and didn't make it, who should have been here today, but they aren't. Because not enough people know about donating. And that's what all this here, this week, has been about—donating."

Jimmy held up a donor card and told everyone there to go home that night and talk to the people who mattered to them about organ donation. And then later in his speech he came back to heroes. "But I have some real special heroes," he said. "Real special people in my life that I look up to and admire and I guess you'd say inspire me. Al Moore is one of those heroes. He's not my brother, least ways not my blood brother, but my spiritual brother maybe, and he's s'posed to be here today, but he's back in Vanderbilt Hospital with rejection, which is something we all have to live with. This day is for him, too.

"And then there's somebody else who was s'posed to be here and couldn't make it, some of y'all maybe know him, but anyway he was a real special man, Mark Johnson. He died a few weeks back in a hunting accident—he was a real keen hunter—and I know he's up in heaven watching us today, and this day's for him, too.

"And, finally, there's the biggest hero of us all. The one who inspired me most to think up this bike trip. Jim Hayes. He's been a heart transplant longer than almost anybody, and he biked all the way across the country once to make people aware. Everybody had given up on him, but not Dr. Frist. And we all know what he has known all along: JIM'S GONNA MAKE IT.

"You know, people who know me, they know I never stop. Soon's I finish one thing, I've got to be doing something else. And everybody's asking me, 'Okay, Jimmy. What are you going to do next?' Well, this day is for Jim Hayes, too, so I want to say today that next year, next year, we're going to bicycle plumb across the whole United States!"

Amid the cheers of the crowd, Karyn looked at me, tears in her eyes.

"Trouble is," I said to her, "he means it."

* * *

263

They were such resilient people, my chimeras. Each and every one of them had said to me at one time or another that they saw life differently now, they understood its value, they wanted to live each moment for what it was, exciting or calm, interesting or boring, aware of all of it, each moment transcendent or mundane. It was a good way to live, much better than the functional lifestyle that was all I could claim for them medically. On the flight home that night with Karyn, I vowed privately that I would live like that too, spend more time with her, with the boys, no matter what the costs, even if I had to give up transplantation to do it. And that night, for sure, I was staying home.

And, for once, I did. Harrison had seen Barbara Mandrell on television that night with Jonathan Jones in a news interview about the upcoming softball game.

"Interview me!" he shouted. "Interview me!"

I picked up a fork and spoke into it. "I'm here with young William Harrison Frist, Jr., to conduct a special in-depth interview on the rare occasion of both his father and mother being home at the same time before his bedtime. Harrison, what does your daddy do?"

Harrison grew stiff, which he equated with becoming adult, and as his mother collapsed, exhausted, into a laughing jag, he said sententiously, "He helps patients."

"What does he do?"

"He takes care."

"What is a transplant?"

"When you help people."

"Do I make them feel better?"

"Yes. You put a new heart in them."

"And where did I get the heart?"

"Out of another person."

"And why did we have to put a new heart in Jonathan Jones?"

"Because his wasn't working."

"Did he have a sick heart?"

"Yes."

"And do you remember meeting Jonathan?"

"Yes."
"Did he look good?"
"Yes. He looked good on TV."

Chuck Norris reminded me of Harrison. He stood there in front of the news camera, his hands behind his back, shifting his weight on his feet uneasily, a shorter man than you would ever imagine from his movies, answering questions about why he was in Nashville to play softball with a bunch of other celebrities for the benefit of heart transplantation.

Behind him, some of the crowd gathered round his fellow notables of stage and screen. Others ate hot dogs, popcorn, and tacos from the mock stands that lined the room or stood, drinks in hand, talking to people they saw every day at work. The reception at the Vanderbilt Plaza Hotel was splendid, well worth the hundred bucks it cost the local doctors, lawyers, businessmen, socialites, and politicos to come and meet the stars.

A set of bleachers off to the right dominated the room. That's where the famous members of each team would sit later for a few minutes while Barbara's husband Ken introduced each of them and while Barbara and Bob Hope held a pep rally of sorts for their troops. Right now most of the entertainers were off in a room upstairs, relaxing, talking to each other, doing whatever they did to get ready to meet the public.

A few opted to join the crowd downstairs and mingle a bit with Nashville's leading citizens or hold impromptu press conferences with the local reporters, all of whom had been carefully cleared at the doors to make sure they belonged. You could tell the stars by their softball uniforms—and by the whispering going on around them. ("Isn't that the Steelers great Lynn Swann?" "L. L. Cool J, or is it J. J. Cool?" "Herschel Walker? *The* Herschel Walker?") Barbara was there, of course, working the crowd well, calling me here to meet this person, walking me there to talk to that one. ("She's so . . . ," Karyn said. "No-nonsense," I offered. "Down-home," the girl from Lubbock replied.) And Barbara's sisters, Irlene and Louise, put in an appearance, along with Sheena Easton, with her sexy, singsong Scottish accent. ("Like two exquisitely chiseled little bookends," I heard one of the city's prominent businessmen say, sipping on his cocktail and eyeing Sheena E. and Louise as they talked with Harvey Bender.)

Dad was there, his fine old features bobbing a head above most of the crowd, enjoying himself immensely, doing what he loved most—visiting those he knew and meeting those he didn't. I hunted him down just before the pep rally was due to begin. Karyn had left to fetch the babysitter, who was upstairs in one of the Plaza's spare rooms, to have her bring the boys down for the finale. I put Harrison up on my shoulders as the rest of the stars— Dick Clark, John Stamos, the heartthrob of the "Full House" television show, Ron Perlman (whom Harrison did not recognize out of his costume from "Beauty and the Beast"), rock musician Meat Loaf, Ralph Emery, Frank Gifford, Emmanuel Lewis, Walter Payton, Minnie Pearl, Ahmad Rashad, Phylicia Rashad, Danny White, Erma Bombeck, the Statler Brothers, Betty White, Oprah Winfrey and, finally, Bob Hope—came out.

The rally consisted mostly of a few showbiz insults and a laying down of the rules of the game, which amounted to one rule: be funny. Afterward, we filed out of the Vanderbilt Plaza and into our various cars and taxis and limos and headed off to join the 25,000 others at the Vanderbilt Stadium.

I found myself on the way over thinking again about celebrity, about all the planning that had gone into this and all the motives behind it, and about the stars themselves. It had been difficult for Barbara to get some of these stars to Nashville, I knew, and I appreciated everything they were doing to help not just me and my patients, but future transplants as well.

In the end, stardom was defined for me not by the Bob Hopes and the Barbara Mandrells, but by the tiny, tiny little black kid down there whom Barbara was leading out to the pitcher's mound as the crowd around us leaned forward in their seats and surged against the rails. And, I thought, it had been difficult for me, too, to get my star here.

We had struggled with a deadly disease, the inadequacies of our social-welfare and health-care systems, the high cost of the only treatment that could save him, an imperfect definition of brain death, the reluctance of doctors to ask survivors to donate, the anger and grief of a family over the tragic loss of a child, the ignorance of the American public about the need for transplantable organs, the shortcomings of our medical technology in organ preservation, immunosuppression, and long-term prognosis, and even my own doubts. In short, we had fought time and nature and society and the unknown to make sure that Jonathan Jones could walk out onto that mound tonight.

Now he stood there, two years old, the same age and with the same name as one of my own sons, the round white softball huge in his small hands. He reared back his arm as Barbara Mandrell stood a few feet in front of him coaching him along. And then he let fly and the crowd roared. The game was on.

The last page of the Vanderbilt University Medical Center report on patient Jim Ray Hayes for the following Monday read in part:

PAGE 3

for continued postoperative care. On FEB 24 the patient was transferred back to the SICU for treatment with OKT3. At this time the patient's endocardial biopsy showed moderate rejection. During this OKT3 treatment, the patient had temperature spikes to 105 degrees. These were treated symptomatically and no cultures were positive. The patient was transferred back to the Seven North Step Down Unit after his OKT3 treatment was finished. On MAR 18 the patient was transferred to the Cooperative Care Unit for continued treatment. On MAR 24, the patient began total lymphoid irradiation to help suppress his moderate transplant rejection. . . . The patient's total lymphoid irradiation was continued until his discharge. A remarkable response. The patient was discharged in excellent condition on JUN 6 to his home in Knoxville, Tennessee.